Alcohol Research
from Bench to Bedside

The *Advances in Alcohol & Substance Abuse* series:

- *Opiate Receptors, Neurotransmitters, & Drug Dependence: Basic Science-Clinical Correlates*
- *Recent Advances in the Biology of Alcoholism*
- *The Effects of Maternal Alcohol and Drug Abuse on the Newborn*
- *Evaluation of Drug Treatment Programs*
- *Current Controversies in Alcoholism*
- *Federal Priorities in Funding Alcohol and Drug Abuse Programs*
- *Psychosocial Constructs of Alcoholism and Substance Abuse*
- *The Addictive Behaviors*
- *Conceptual Issues in Alcoholism and Substance Abuse*
- *Dual Addiction: Pharmacological Issues in the Treatment of Concomitant Alcoholism and Drug Abuse*
- *Cultural and Sociological Aspects of Alcoholism and Substance Abuse*
- *Alcohol and Drug Abuse in the Affluent*
- *Alcohol and Substance Abuse in Adolescence*
- *Controversies in Alcoholism and Substance Abuse*
- *Alcohol and Substance Abuse in Women and Children*
- *Cocaine: Pharmacology, Addiction, and Therapy*
- *Children of Alcoholics*
- *Pharmacological Issues in Alcohol and Substance Abuse*
- *AIDS and Substance Abuse*
- *Alcohol Research from Bench to Bedside*

Alcohol Research from Bench to Bedside

Guest Editors
Enoch Gordis, MD
Boris Tabakoff, PhD
Markku Linnoila, MD, PhD
Editor
Barry Stimmel, MD

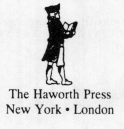

The Haworth Press
New York • London

Alcohol Research from Bench to Bedside has also been published as *Advances in Alcohol & Substance Abuse*, Volume 7, Numbers 3/4 1988.

The Haworth Press, Inc., 12 West 32 Street, New York, NY 10001
EUROSPAN/Haworth, 3 Henrietta Street, London WC2E 8LU England

Library of Congress Cataloging-in-Publication Data

Alcohol research from bench to bedside / guest editors, Enoch Gordis, Boris Tabakoff, Markku Linnoila ; editor, Barry Stimmel.
    p. cm.
    "Has also been published as Advances in alcohol & substance abuse, volume 7, number 3/4 1988" — T.p. verso.
    Based on a symposium held in 1987 at the National Institutes of Health in Bethesda, Md. and sponsored by the National Institute on Alcohol Abuse and Alcoholism.
    Includes bibliographies.
    ISBN 0-86656-852-2
    1. Alcoholism — Congresses. 2. Alcohol — Health aspects — Congresses. I. Gordis, Enoch, 1931- . II. Tabakoff, B. (Boris) III. Linnoila, Markku. IV. National Institute on Alcohol Abuse and Alcoholism (U.S.)
    [DNLM: 1. Alcohol, Ethyl — pharmacology — congresses. 2. Alcoholism — congresses. 3. Research — United States — congresses. W1 AD432 v. 7 no. 3/4 / WM 274 A35275 1987]
RC565.A4444   1988
616.86'1 — dc19
DNLM/DLC
for Library of Congress   88-30140
                                                          CIP

Alcohol Research from Bench to Bedside

CONTENTS

NEUROSCIENCE AND PSYCHOPHARMACOLOGY

ABOUT THE GUEST EDITORS

Enoch Gordis, MD, has been the Director of the National Institute on Alcohol Abuse and Alcoholism (NIAAA) since October, 1986. Prior to this, he directed the alcoholism program at Elmhurst Hospital in Elmhurst, New York for 15 years, and was Professor of Clinical Medicine at Mt. Sinai School of Medicine in New York City. A recognized expert on alcoholism treatment, Dr. Gordis has written extensively on a variety of alcohol-related research and clinical topics including treatment outcome research, ethanol and methadone drug interactions, disulfiram therapy in alcoholism, and alcoholism and drug addiction in pregnancy.

Boris Tabakoff, PhD, is Director of the Intramural Research Program, Division of Intramural Clinical and Biological Research of the National Institute on Alcohol Abuse and Alcoholism (NIAAA). Dr. Tabakoff was trained as a molecular pharmacologist and also received training in behavioral genetics. His research has resulted in over 170 published papers. Dr. Tabakoff came to the NIAAA from the University of Illinois Medical Center, where he was Professor of Physiology and Biophysics, as well as the Director of the Alcohol and Drug Abuse Research and Training Program.

Markku Linnoila, MD, PhD, is Clinical Director, Division of Intramural Clinical and Biological Research, National Institute on Alcohol Abuse and Alcoholism (NIAAA). He is also on the Psycho-pharmacologic Drugs Advisory Committee of the Food and Drug Administration, and is Cochairman, Secretary of HSS Task Force on Youth Suicide, Working Group on Risk Factors. His previous positions included Staff Psychiatrist at the National Institute of Mental Health, and until 1987, Dr. Linnoila was affiliated with Duke University Medical Center as Associate Professor of Psychiatry and of Pharmacology, as well as Head of the Clinical Psychopharmacology Section. Dr. Linnoila received his graduate degrees from the University of Helsinki, Finland, where he occasionally returns to teach pharmacology.

Alcohol Research
from Bench to Bedside

EDITORIAL

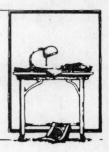

During 1987, the National Institutes of Health (NIH) celebrated their 100th anniversary. A large number of events were held on the NIH campus in Bethesda, Maryland, and throughout the world, to mark this occasion.

The Alcohol Drug Abuse and Mental Health Administration (ADAMHA), which has programs on the NIH campus, joined in the commemoration activities. As part of the NIH 100th anniversary celebration, the National Institute on Alcohol Abuse and Alcoholism (NIAAA), one of the ADAMHA Institutes, sponsored a Symposium entitled, "Alcohol Research from Bench to Bedside." This Symposium helped to focus attention on the 100 years of science supported by the Federal government. These endeavors in science have produced medical knowledge applicable to a wide spectrum of treatment and prevention efforts. The Symposium brought together basic scientists and clinicians whose work on alcohol's actions and alcoholism was presented through lectures, as well as poster presentations. These printed proceedings contain the record of much of what was discussed during the Symposium.

The Symposium also served as a tribute to the collaborations that have developed between NIAAA Intramural researchers and other researchers at NIH. Ongoing collaborative ventures with scientists in neurology, child health, digestive diseases, and even dentistry, have enhanced the opportunities to apply the latest technology and the latest medical knowledge to studies of alcohol's actions and alcoholism. On the other hand, the various clinical and basic science research programs at NIH have benefited from the NIAAA scientists' expertise on alcoholism within the context of numerous health related projects. The "Alcohol Research from Bench to Bedside" Symposium also allowed for highlighting the symbiotic relationships established between the alcoholism treatment community throughout the country and the NIAAA Intramural researchers. The all-day meeting was attended by well over 400 registrants, many of whom were treatment and prevention professionals.

As can be seen from the text of the many papers that make up these proceedings, the topics ranged in scope from studies on the molecular actions of alcohol to clinical studies with human subjects. Alcoholism is a complex, multi-faceted syndrome, with both biological and environmental determinants contributing to the etiology of the disorder. Not until science develops an understanding of both the biological/genetic and the environmental mechanisms underlying alcoholism, can definitive treatment and prevention approaches be instituted. The need to understand alcoholism at all levels of biologic and social complexity provides enormous opportunities for collaboration between bench and bedside scientists. It is hoped that published proceedings of the "Alcohol Research from Bench to Bedside" Symposium, sponsored by NIAAA, will enhance the communication of ideas between all segments of the research and treatment communities and will catalyze progress in eliminating the damage that alcohol causes in our society.

Enoch Gordis, MD, Director, NIAAA
Boris Tabakoff, PhD, Scientific Director, NIAAA
Markku Linnoila, MD, PhD, Clinical Director, NIAAA

ACKNOWLEDGEMENTS

The Editors wish to acknowledge the superb assistance provided by Benedict Latteri, in organizing the Symposium, *Alcohol Research from Bench to Bedside*; and the editorial assistance of Nancy Yellin, without whose help the publication of these Proceedings would not have been possible.

Genetic Heterogeneity
and the Classification of Alcoholism

C. Robert Cloninger, MD
Soren Sigvardsson, PhD
Shelia B. Gilligan, BS
Anna-Liis von Knorring, MD
Theodore Reich, MD
Michael Bohman, MD

SUMMARY. Recent progress toward a systematic pathophysiological model of alcoholism has led to identification of two distinct subtypes of alcoholism. These subtypes may be distinguished in terms of distinct alcohol-related symptoms, personality traits, ages of onset, and patterns of inheritance. Type 1 alcoholism is characterized by anxious (passive-dependent) personality traits and rapid development of tolerance and dependence on the anti-anxiety effects of alco-

C. Robert Cloninger, Shelia B. Gilligan, and Theodore Reich are affiliated with the Departments of Psychiatry & Genetics, Washington University, School of Medicine and Jewish Hospital, 216 South Kingshighway Blvd., St. Louis, MO 63110. Soren Sigvardsson, Anna-Liis von Knorring, and Michael Bohman are affiliated with the Department of Child & Youth Psychiatry, Umea University, Sweden. Reprint requests should be addressed to C. Robert Cloninger.

This project was supported in part by NIAAA grant AA-03539, NIMH Research Scientist Award MG-00048, and Swedish Medical Research Council grant B85-25X-06368-04C.

hol. This leads to loss of control, difficulty terminating binges once they start, guilt feelings, and liver complications following socially encouraged exposure to alcohol intake. In contrast, type 2 alcoholism is characterized by antisocial personality traits and persistent seeking of alcohol for its euphoriant effects. This leads to early onset of inability to abstain entirely, as well as fighting and arrests when drinking. Empirical findings about sex differences, ages of onset, associated personality traits, and longitudinal course are described in a series of adoption and family studies in Sweden and the United States. Implications for future research and clinical practice are discussed.

Recent family and adoption studies have identified subtypes of alcoholics who differ in alcohol-related symptoms, personality traits, and pattern of inheritance.[1-5] Many past studies had treated alcoholism as if it were a single discrete entity despite the repeated observation that core symptoms of dependence, social problems, family problems, and depressive symptoms are only weakly correlated with one another.[6] Also alcoholism is associated with antisocial personality traits in some families, but not others.[5,7,8] Similarly, antisocial traits are characteristic of most alcoholics with onset in adolescence or early adulthood, but only a minority of those with later onset.[9] In contrast, passive-dependent personality traits have been found to increase the risk of later alcoholism in some, but not all, longitudinal studies.[10] Hence alcoholism appears to be heterogeneous in its causes, course, and clinical features.

Findings about the inheritance of alcoholism and related disorders have been instrumental in defining current approaches to the classification of alcoholic subtypes. Progress in defining different types of alcoholism will be described by describing the actual sequence of research results obtained in collaborative studies carried out in Sweden and the United States. Key findings of clinical or etiological importance will be emphasized.

STOCKHOLM ADOPTION STUDY

Michael Bohman and his associates in Sweden initiated a large scale study of all adopted children who had been born to single women in Stockholm from 1930 to 1949. Eight hundred and sixty-two men and 913 women of known paternity who had been adopted by nonrelatives before 3 years of age were identified. Most of the adoptees were separated from their biological relatives in the first few months of life, and the average age at separation was 4 months.[1-3] Information about alcohol abuse, psychopathology, and medical treatment was available for the entire lifetimes of the adoptees and their parents (adoptive and biological) from hospitals, clinics, and several registers that are systematically maintained in Sweden. Identification of alcohol abuse using these sources has been found to identify about 70% of alcoholics.[11] Alcoholics identified in this way are representative of alcoholics in general, having no significant differences in personality disorders or traits when compared to other alcoholics.[12] Hence adoptees and their parents were identified as alcohol abusers if they were ever registered with the Swedish Temperance Boards for alcohol abuse, treated for alcoholism in hospitals or clinics, or diagnosed as alcoholic by a psychiatrist.

Professor Bohman viewed the adoption situation as an opportunity to reverse the negative social heritage of the adoptees, whose biological parents often had low socioeconomic status and a higher frequency of alcohol abuse than in the general population (32.4% of 1775 biological fathers, 4.7% of 1775 biological mothers). In fact, the risk of alcohol abuse in the adoptees (17.5% of 862 men, 3.4% of 913 women) was about half that of their fathers, but such differences between generations may be attributable to a variety of secular changes. In fact, alcohol abuse in the adoptive parents was not associated with an increased risk of alcohol abuse in the adoptees, suggesting that imitation of parental drinking is not a major determinant of alcohol abuse.[1,2]

In contrast, alcohol abuse in the biological parents was associated with a substantial increased risk of alcohol abuse in their adopted-away children. The risk of alcohol abuse was studied in the children when they were 23 to 43 years of age. As shown in Table 1, the adopted-away sons were more likely to be alcohol abusers if either their biological father or mother had been registered for alcohol abuse than if neither parent had been registered for alcohol abuse. However, the adopted-away daughters were more likely to be alcohol abusers only if their biological mother had been registered for alcohol abuse, not if neither parent or only the biological father had

Table 1

Inheritance of Susceptibility to Alcohol Abuse
in the Stockholm Adoption Study

Alcohol abuse in biological parents		Alcohol abuse in adoptees			
		Sons		Daughters	
Father	Mother	N	%	N	%
No	No	571	14.7	577	2.8
Yes	No	259	22.4	285	3.5
No	Yes	23	26.0	29	10.3
Yes	Yes	9	33.3	22	9.1

been registered for alcohol abuse. This sex difference suggested that some types of alcohol abuse might be heritable primarily in men; whereas, other forms may be heritable in both men and women.[1,2]

Cross-Fostering Analysis of Adopted Men

In order to evaluate the inheritance of heterogeneous groups of alcohol abusers, the adopted men were subdivided according to their frequency and severity of registered abuse, as suggested by Kaij based on detailed personal assessments.[13] Specifically, we distinguished adopted men who had "mild abuse" (only single registrations with the Temperance Board and no treatment), "moderate abuse" (two or three registrations and no treatment), and "severe abuse" (treatment for alcoholism, psychiatric diagnosis of alcoholism, or more than three registrations with the Temperance Board). The biological parents[1,13] of the moderate abusers ("type 2") were found to differ significantly from those of the parents of the other ("type 1") abusers; their fathers more often had teenage onset of both criminal behavior and severe alcohol abuse. In contrast, the biological fathers of the type 1 alcohol abusers usually had later adult onset of mild alcohol abuse without associated criminal behavior; this was true whether the severity of abuse in the adoptee was mild or severe. Furthermore, the biological mothers of the type 1 alcohol abusers had a substantial increased risk of alcohol abuse: whereas, the biological mothers of the type 2 alcohol abusers had no excess compared to the mothers of nonalcoholic adoptees. The only observed differences in the backgrounds of the mild and severe type 1 alcohol abusers was in the occupational status of their biological and adoptive parents; severe abuse was more likely to occur in those with predisposition to low occupational status, which was in turn associated with heavier recreational drinking. These findings suggested that there were genetic differences between type 1 and type 2 alcohol abusers, but not between mild and severe type 1 alcohol abusers. In other words, the differences between mild and severe alcohol abusers were largely determined by environmental exposure variables, not genetic factors.

The importance of postnatal environmental factors on severity of type 1 alcohol abuse was examined in a cross-fostering analysis of the 862 adopted men. In a cross-fostering analysis, the risk of disorder in adoptees is considered as a consequence of different combinations of biological parent background and postnatal environmental experience. This is illustrated in Table 2 for alcohol abuse in the 862 adopted men. The risk of severe abuse doubled in sons who had both type 1 biological parents (as described above) and low occupational status in their adoptive home. Likewise the risk of mild abuse depended on both the genetic and the environmental background. Accordingly, type 1 alcoholism has also been called "milieu-limited" alcoholism.

In contrast, type 2 alcoholism was highly heritable from father to son regardless of external circumstances (Table 3). The risk in sons of type 2 fathers was increased about nine-fold compared to the risk in other fathers, including those with either type 1 or no alcoholism.

Cross-Fostering Analysis of Adopted Women

Next we carried out tests of predictions in adopted women in order to test the validity of the type 1 and type 2 distinction that we had developed in the studies of the adopted men.[2,3] First, we had predicted that type 1, but not type 2, biological parents would have an excess of adopted-away daughters with alcohol abuse. This prediction was based on the finding that mothers of type 1 alcoholics had often been alcoholics, but not those of type 2 alcoholics.

To carry out the test of this prediction we classified the biological

Table 2

Cross-fostering Analysis of Mild and
Severe Type 1 Alcoholism

Is Genetic Background Type 1?	Is Environmental Background Mild or Severe?	Male Adoptees Observed		
		Total N	% With Mild Abuse	% With Severe Abuse
No	–	448	6.5	42.
Yes	No	237	7.2	6.3
Yes	Mild	91	15.4*	7.7
Yes	Severe	86	4.7	11.6*

*Abuse is increased only given both genetic and postnatal predispositon (P<.05).

Table 3

Cross-Fostering Analysis of Type 2 Alcohol Abuse in Men

Is genetic background type 2?	Is environmental background type 2?	Male adoptees observed	
		Total N	% with type 2 abuse
No	No	567	1.9
No	Yes	196	4.1
Yes	No	71	16.9[a]
Yes	Yes	28	17.9[a]

[a] Risk is significantly increased in thos with type 2 genetic background compared to others (P<0.01).

parents of the adopted women using a multivariate discriminant function derived from the male sample. That is, we classified the biological parents of the women according to several characteristics that had distinguished the subgroups of male alcoholics, such as age of onset of alcohol abuse and associated criminality. Thus we classified the biological parent backgrounds in exactly the same way regardless of the sex of the adoptee. Then we checked to see what behaviors were actually observed in the adopted women. The behaviors of daughters of type 1 and type 2 biological families are summarized in Tables 4 and 5 respectively. As predicted, the type 1 daughters were more likely to be alcohol abusers than were type 2 or other daughters.

Furthermore, we found that the type 2 daughters were likely to have prominent somatization as evidence by their excessive physical complaints and sick leave disability.[14] In particular, the type 2 daughters had frequent and diverse physical complaints, such as headaches, backaches, and stomachaches. This was consistent with other studies that had observed an association of Briquet's syndrome or somatization disorder in men with antisocial personality and alcoholism in men in the same family. In other words, given the same genetic predisposition, men usually express type 2 alcoholism and women usually express somatization. Somatization in women and type 2 alcoholism in men are associated with antisocial personality traits.[15]

PERSONALITY AND ALCOHOLISM SUBTYPES

In addition, it was possible to identify men and women at high risk for alcoholism by selection of adoptees with different forms of anxiety of somatization. Cognitive anxiety refers to frequent anticipatory worrying associated with complaints of weakness and fatigue, but infrequent headaches, backaches, and other bodily complaints. Cognitive anxiety is associated with passive-dependent personality traits, including (i) high harm avoidance (that is, cautious, apprehensive, pessimistic, inhibited, shy, and fatigable), (ii) high reward dependence (that is, eager to help others, emotionally dependent, warmly sympathetic, sentimental, sensitive to social cues, and persistent), and (iii) low novelty seeking (that is, rigid, reflective, loyal, orderly, and attentive to details). In contrast, individuals with somatic anxiety or somatization have the reverse configuration of personality traits, which is characteristic of antisocial personality, including (i) low harm avoidance (that is, confident, relaxed, optimistic, uninhibited, carefree, and energetic) (ii) high novelty seeking (that is, impulsive, exploratory, excitable, disorderly, and distractible) (iii) low reward dependence (that is, socially detached, emotionally cool, practical, tough-minded, and independently self-willed). Individuals with either cognitive or somatic anxiety were at increased

Table 4

Psychopathology in the Adopted-out Daughters of Type 1
Biologic Parents and of Nonalcoholic Biologic Parents

Observed psychopathology[b]	Classification of daughters[a]		
	Type 1 (N = 110) row %	Low risk (N = 282) row %	Significance level P
Alcohol abuse	7.3	2.5	<0.05[c]
Criminality only	0	1.4	NS
Somatization only	16.3	16.3	NS
Other disability	13.6	15.2	NS

[a] Classification of the biologic parents of the women was based on discriminant analysis of an independent sample of parents of adopted men.

[b] The classification system for adoptees was hierarchical, proceeding from alcohol abuse to other psychiatric disability. Thus criminality only indicates criminality and no alcohol abuse with or without somatization or other disability; somatization only indicates neither alcohol abuse nor criminality.

[c] Risk is increased compared with low-risk daughters.

risk for alcoholism. However, adoptees with cognitive anxiety had fewer criminal biological parents than in the general population (as expected for type 1 alcoholism). Also adoptees with somatic anxiety had more criminal biological parents than in the general population (as expected for type 2 alcoholism).

In order to test the proposed role of personality in the development of alcoholism, we carried out a prospective longitudinal study of 431 schoolchildren in Sweden.[9] The personality and behavioral adjustment of the children had been assessed when they were 10 to 11 years of age by a detailed interview of their teachers. This permitted rating of the three dimensions of personality (harm avoidance, novelty seeking, and reward dependence) independent of any other information about their later behavior. Independently, records about alcohol abuse were obtained through the age of 27 years. We predicted that such early-onset alcohol abuse would be primarily type 2 alcoholism associated with antisocial personality traits (low harm avoidance, high novelty seeking, and low reward depen-

Table 5

Psychopathology in the Adopted-out Daughters of Type 2
Biologic Parents and of Nonalcoholic Biologic Parents

| Observed Psychopathology[b] | Classification of daughters[a] | | Significance level P |
	Type 2 (N = 105) row %	Low risk (N = 282) row %	
Alcohol Abuse	4.8	2.5	NS
Criminality Only	2.9	1.4	NS
Somatization Only	26.7	16.3	<0.05[c]
Other Disability	13.3	15.2	NS

[a] Classification of the biologic parents of the women was based on discriminant analysis of an independent sample of parents of adopted men.

[b] The classification system for adoptees was hierachical, proceeding from alcohol abuse to other psychiatric disability. Thus criminality only indicates criminality and no alcohol abuse with or without somatization or other disability; somatization only indicates neither alcohol abuse nor criminality.

[c] Risk is increased compared with low-risk daughters.

dence), even though some type 1 alcoholics might be present also. In other words, average personality traits were expected to be associated with the lowest risk of alcoholism. These expectations were confirmed, as summarized in Table 6, about the 233 men. Logistic regression analysis revealed that childhood ratings of novelty seeking, harm avoidance, and reward dependence distinguished groups of boys who differed in their risk of alcohol abuse from 4% to 75%.

ST. LOUIS FAMILY STUDY

In order to obtain more detailed descriptions of the two types of alcoholism, we carried out pedigree analyses of families of 286 hospitalized alcoholics studied in St. Louis as part of the Washington University Alcoholism Research Center since 1977. Direct interview data were available for 176 male first-degree relatives of

Table 6

Quantitative Personality Deviation and Non-Linearity
of Risk for Later Alcohol Abuse

Childhood Personality Rating	# Boys	% Alcohol Abuse	Risk Ratio*
Harm Avoidance			
+2 or +3	21	14	1.6
+1	49	8	0.9
0	99	9	1.0
-1	39	18	2.0
-2 or -3	25	28	3.1
Novelty Seeking			
+2 or +3	65	25	2.3
+1	24	4	0.4
0	101	11	1.0
-1	27	0	0.0
-2 or -3	16	13	1.2
Reward Dependence			
+2 or +3	30	20	2.5
+1	67	12	1.5
0	89	8	1.0
-1	29	17	2.2
-2 or -3	18	22	2.8

* Risk ratio is the ratio of the risk in the specified group to the risk of average individuals.

male probands and 67 male relatives of female probands.[15] First, we identified the alcohol-related symptoms that best distinguished men in the families of female probands from men in the families of male probands. The distinguishing characteristics of men according to the sex of the proband are summarized in Table 7. The type 2 syndrome, which is characteristic of men in families of male alcoholics, is distinguished by individuals with onset of persistent alcohol-seeking behavior ("inability to abstain entirely") before age 25 years, fights while drinking, arrests for reckless driving while drinking, and treatment for alcohol abuse.

In contrast, the type 1 syndrome, which is characteristic of men related to female alcoholics, is distinguished by onset after age 25 years of loss of control, guilt feelings, binges, and liver disease. After regression on the total number of alcoholic symptoms, the residual numbers of type 1 and type 2 symptoms were negatively

Table 7

Alcohol-related Symptoms Distinguishing Male
Relatives of Female Probands From Male Probands

Distinguishing characteristics of male relatives[1]	Discriminant coefficient	Variable means of relatives by sex of proband	
		Male proband (N = 176)	Female proband (N = 67)
Type 1 features			
benders	+0.55	0.16	0.22
guilt	+0.45	0.20	0.30
onset after 25[2]	+0.40	0.18	0.30
loss of control	+0.33	0.25	0.30
cirrhosis/liver disease	+0.25	0.20	0.06
Type 2 features			
inability to abstain	-0.23	0.19	0.15
fights while drinking	-0.44	0.42	0.24
reckless driving while drinking	-0.45	0.32	0.20
treatment for alcohol abuse	-0.46	0.11	0.06
Discriminant function score	---	-0.24	+0.62
Number of alcoholic symptoms[3]			
type 1	---	1.1	2.0
type 2	---	1.0	0.6

[1] Variables were selected by stepwise discriminant function analysis (total explained variance = 12.8%, Wilk's λ = 0.872, p = 0.0002).

[2] Denotes the proportion of relatives with age at onset of second alcohol-related problem after 25 years of age.

[3] After regression on the total number of Feighner alcoholic symptoms, the residual numbers of type 1 and type 2 symptoms were negatively correlated in male relatives (r = -0.23).

correlated in male relatives (r = -0.23), as expected from their relationship to opposite personality traits.

Pedigree analyses were also carried out to evaluate heterogeneity among the male alcoholics. The families of male alcoholics were highly heterogeneous, some having patterns more like the families of female alcoholics (that is, type 1 alcoholic men) and others having inheritance patterns like the families of men only (that is, type 2 alcoholic men). For example, heritability of alcoholism in type 2 families was 88%, and that in type 1 families was 21%,[5] estimates similar to those obtained in the Stockholm Adoption Study.[1] Accordingly, findings initially obtained in Swedish families have been replicated in American families.

DISCUSSION

This series of adoption and family studies has defined a consistent set of distinguishing characteristics for two subgroups of alcoholics. The distinguishing features are summarized in Table 8. Type 1 alcoholics have personality traits that make them susceptible to anxiety; in response to the anti-anxiety effects of alcohol, they rapidly become tolerant and dependent and have difficulty terminating drinking binges once they have started ("loss of control"). Type 2 alcoholics have antisocial personality traits; they persistently seek alcohol for its euphoriant effects ("inability to abstain").[16]

These differences in clinical features and patterns of inheritance are associated with other neurophysiological and psychopharmacological differences summarized elsewhere.[4] For example, abstinent type 1 alcoholics have minimal brain-wave activity in the slow al-

Table 8

Distinguishing Characteristics of Two Types of Alcoholism

Characteristic Features	Type of Alcoholism	
	Type 1	Type 2
Alcohol-related problems		
Usual age of onset (years)	Ater 25	Before 25
Spontaneous alcohol-seeking (inability to abstain)	Infrequent	Frequent
Fighting and arrests when drinking	Infrequent	Frequent
Psychological dependence (loss of control)	Frequent	Infrequent
Guilt and fear about (alcohol dependence)	Frequent	Infrequent
Personality Traits		
Novelty seeking	Low	High
Harm avoidance	High	Low
Reward dependence	High	Low

pha frequency range, excessive beta activity, and poor synchrony.[17] In contrast, abstinent type 2 alcoholics and their sons have augmenting perceptual reactance to stimulation of increasing intensity, as well as a reduced amplitude of the late positive component (P3) of the event-related brain-wave potential.[18]

A general model of the neurogenetic basis of personality that accounts for available information about susceptibility to alcoholism and related disorders has been presented elsewhere.[4,19] This general model is supported by extensive experimental data in rodents, as described in part by results presented by Dr. Li elsewhere in this volume. In addition, supporting neurochemical data in humans is available. Type 1 alcoholics with loss of control and craving for alcohol have lower basal noradrenergic activity after several months of abstinence than other alcoholics.[20] In contrast, abstinent type 2 alcoholics with prominent impulsive-aggressive behavior have low levels of serotonergic and dopaminergic metabolites in their cerebrospinal fluid,[4] as discussed by Dr. Linnoila elsewhere in this volume.

Despite the differences among type 1 and type 2 alcoholics, there is still often overlap in symptoms, particularly in treatment samples. Our results suggest that two opposing processes predispose to alcohol abuse, not that there are two discrete entities. Risk of alcoholism is a quantitative variable, not a dichotomy or trichotomy. A brief 100-item self-report inventory called the Tridimensional Personality Questionnaire (TPQ) has been developed to measure the relevant personality traits,[19] and is available for research purposes. Accordingly, researchers are encouraged to make quantitative ratings of personality variables that can be related to other variables. Likewise, clinicians are encouraged to make quantitative assessments that can be used in planning prevention and treatment efforts.

REFERENCES

1. Cloninger CR, Bohman M, Sigvardsson S. Inheritance of alcohol abuse: cross-fostering analysis of adopted men. Arch Gen Psychiatry 1981; 38:861-868.

2. Bohman M, Sigvardsson S, Cloninger CR. Maternal inheritance of alcohol abuse: cross-fostering analysis of adopted women. Arch Gen Psychiatry 1981; 38:965-969.

3. Cloninger CR, Bohman M, Sigvardsson S, von Knorring A-L. Psychopathology in adopted-out children of alcoholics: the Stockholm adoption study. Recent Developments in Alcoholism 1985; 3:37-51.

4. Cloninger CR. Neurogenetic adaptive mechanisms in alcoholism. Science 1987; 236:410-416.

5. Gilligan SB, Reich T, Cloninger CR. Etiologic heterogeneity in alcoholism. Genetic Epidemiology 1987; in press.

6. Park P, Whitehead P. Developmental sequence and dimensions of alcoholism. Quart J Stud Alcohol 1973; 34:887-904.

7. Cloninger CR, Reich T, Wetzel R. Alcoholism and affective disorders: familial associations and genetic models. In: Goodwin D, Erickson C, eds. Alcoholism and Affective Disorders. New York, Spectrum Press, 1979, pp. 57-86.

8. Cloninger CR, Reich T. Genetic heterogeneity in alcoholism and sociopathy. In: Kety SS, Rowland LP, Sidman RL, Matthyssee SW, eds. Genetics of Neurological and Psychiatric Disorders. New York, Raven Press, 1983, pp. 145-165.

9. Cloninger CR, Sigvardsson S, Bohman M. Childhood personality predicts alcohol abuse in young adults. Alcoholism: Clinical & Experimental Research, in press.

10. Block J. Lives Through Time. Berkeley, California, Bancroft Books, 1971.

11. Ojesjo L. Prevalence of known and hidden alcoholism in the revisited Lundby population. Social Psychiatry 1980; 15:81-90.

12. Kaij L. Biases in a Swedish social register of alcoholics. Social Psychiatry 1970; 5:216-218.

13. Kaij L. Alcoholism in Twins: Studies on the Etiology and Sequels of Abuse of Alcohol. Stockholm, Almqvist & Wiksell, 1960.

14. Bohman M, Cloninger CR, von Knorring A-L, Sigvardsson S. An adoption study of somatoform disorders. III. cross-fostering analysis and genetic relationship to alcoholism and criminality. Arch Gen Psychiatry 1984; 41:872-878.

15. Cloninger CR. A unified biosocial theory of personality and its role in the development of anxiety states. Psychiatric Developments 1986; 3:167-226.

16. Nordstrom G, Berglund M. Different patterns of successful long-term adjustment in genetically defined subtypes of alcoholics. Alcohol & Alcoholism 1987; Suppl 1:401-405.

17. Propping P, Kruger J, Mark N. Hum Genet 1981; 59:51.

18. Begleiter H, Projesz B, Rawlings R, Eckardt M. Auditory recovery function and P3 in boys at high risk for alcoholism. Alcohol 1987; 4:315-321.

19. Cloninger CR. A systematic method for clinical description and classification of personality variants. Arch Gen Psychiatry 1987; 44:573-588.

20. Borg S, Liljeberg P, Mossberg D. Clinical studies on central noradrenergic activity in alcohol abusing patients. Acta Psychiatrica Scand 1986; Suppl 327:43-60.

Neurotransmitters and Alcoholism: Methodological Issues

Markku Linnoila, MD, PhD

SUMMARY. This short review examines recent findings on neurochemical differences between alcoholics and various control populations. Particular emphasis is given to clinical variables which affect concentrations of neurotransmitter metabolites in the cerebrospinal fluid, and which have to be controlled in order to make meaningful comparisons between various diagnostic groups. The review focuses on two of the major monoamine transmitters, serotonin and norepinephrine, and excludes neurotransmitters and modulators such as dopamine, acetylcholine, peptides, prostaglandins, amino acids and purines, since their significance to alcoholism is currently less well understood.

Alcoholism is the most common mental disorder among men in the U.S. with the highest prevalence among the 24 to 40 age group.[1] According to the 3rd edition of the American Psychiatric Association's Diagnostic and Statistical Manual (DSM III[2]), alcoholism is subdivided into alcohol dependence and alcohol abuse. The term alcoholism itself is no longer used in this diagnostic classification. Alcohol dependence and abuse are differentiated from each other by the duration of excessive drinking and the severity of its consequences. The clinical and scientific utility of this differentiation is questionable at the present time.

A more useful classification of patients with alcoholism can probably be accomplished by dividing them into primary and sec-

Markku Linnoila is affiliated with the Laboratory of Clinical Studies, Division of Intramural Clinical and Biological Research, National Institute on Alcohol Abuse and Alcoholism, NIH Clinical Center, Bldg. 10, Rm. 3C218, Bethesda, MD 20892.

17

ondary groups. In primary alcoholics, alcoholism began prior to the onset of any other mental disorder, whereas in secondary alcoholics the onset of another mental disorder preceded the onset of alcoholism. The primary-secondary differentiation has a long tradition. It uses the relative age of onset of the various mental disorders as the distinguishing criterion.[3] Using this simple time of onset criterion more men are classified as primary and more women as secondary alcoholics.[4] This difference partially reflects the later average age of onset of alcoholism in women.[5]

Family and adoption studies on alcoholism have established a powerful genetic contribution to the risk of becoming alcoholic.[6-8] Furthermore, recent large scale adoption studies by Cloninger et al. have demonstrated that there are at least two genetically different types of alcoholism, Type I and Type II.[9] Type I is the more common form of the illness. It affects both men and women. Adverse environmental factors have a strong impact on the expression of the genetic vulnerability, particularly in men. Type II affects about 25% of male alcoholics. The illness is characterized by an early age of onset and the coexistence of antisocial and criminal behaviors in the male members of the families. Environmental contribution to the expression of the inherited vulnerability towards alcoholism is negligible in these patients. This gene effect is not expressed as alcoholism in women. Certain investigators have suggested that men with primary alcoholism often have a history of hyperactivity.[10] Up to 30% of hyperactive boys without a conduct disorder may grow up to have antisocial personality disorder.[11,12] In these individuals, childhood hyperactivity may, therefore, represent an age appropriate expression of the Type II alcoholism gene effect.

For psychobiological studies to meaningfully elucidate pathophysiology and risk factors of any illness requires that homogenous patient groups are compared with appropriate controls. The interpretation of past studies on alcoholism is complicated by the partial overlap of the clinically important primary-secondary dichotomy and the Type I-Type II classification deduced from the adoption study data.

One way to circumvent these difficulties and to achieve relatively homogenous patient groups for biological studies is to use both family history and clinical features of the patient for classification.

According to this scheme the first distinction to be made in a hierarchical diagnostic process would be between Type I and Type II alcoholics. The symptoms of past hyperactivity, antisocial personality disorder, criminality and alcoholism are considered to be expressions of the same genetic vulnerability to Type II alcoholism. Thus, symptoms of hyperactivity, antisocial and criminal behaviors are not used to make a primary-secondary classification in these patients. The main problem for psychobiological research in this group of patients is that in contemporary U.S. metropolitan areas they very often are polysubstance abusers. If polysubstance abusers are included in a sample for psychobiological study, long term effects of drug abuse may erroneously be assumed to be abnormalities characteristic of Type II alcoholism. If, on the other hand, patients with polysubstance abuse are excluded from the sample, its representativeness may be questionable. At the present time, excluding polysubstance users from psychobiological studies on Type II alcoholism is probably the preferable alternative.

After identifying patients with Type II alcoholism, a clear distinction has to be made between primary and secondary alcoholism in the remaining patients. Those with primary alcoholism should be representative of Type I. Secondary alcoholism would be considered to be a complication of a primary mental disorder.

FAMILIAL COMORBIDITY

Alcoholism is more common in families with anxiety disorders, particularly panic disorder and agoraphobia, eating disorders and affective disorder.[13] Making an unequivocal diagnosis of primary versus secondary alcoholism in patients with family histories of any of these disorders, although simple in theory, can be very complicated in practice. This is particularly true when one or both disorders have an insidious onset.

SPECIFIC BEHAVIORS

Psychiatric diagnoses, even when successful in delineating relatively homogenous patient groups, represent descriptions of syndromes. There is no a priori reason why a compilation of symptoms should be related to a biochemical abnormality. Indeed it is more likely that specific behaviors rather than a diagnosis incorporating a variety of abnormal behaviors will be related to specific neurotransmitter functions. The symptom of suicidal behavior is a good example of such a situation. It is robustly associated with indices of reduced central nervous system serotonin metabolism in patients with various mental disorders including alcoholism.[14]

Thus, it is important to quantify specific behaviors using well established rating scales and behavioral inventories once diagnosing and subgrouping patients with alcoholism have been accomplished. These data can be used in addition to the diagnostic subgrouping in search of specific psychobiological correlates of alcoholism.

STATE AND TRAIT

Adverse life events often precede the onset of a mental disorder. Their contribution to the onset of a given mental disorder is, however, nonspecific at best.[15] Moreover, subclinical prodromal symptoms of an oncoming mental disorder may facilitate the occurrence of adverse life events such as separation. Be this as it may, major adverse life events may produce significant state dependent changes in concentrations of neurotransmitter metabolites in various body fluids.[16] Thus, life events have to be carefully recorded and their impact on the life of a given patient should be investigated.

In studies on alcoholism, an important state variable is *alcohol withdrawal*. In most patients, its major symptoms are over after a ten day period of abstinence, but cross-sectional studies suggest that biochemical changes, such as elevated cerebrospinal fluid (CSF) 5-hydroxyindoleacetic acid (5-HIAA) concentration, last a minimum of two to three weeks.[17,18] 5-HIAA is the principal metabolite of serotonin and its concentration in the CSF is often used as an indicator of central nervous system serotonin functioning. Good longitudinal psychobiological studies on the duration of withdrawal induced changes on central nervous system biochemistry are sorely needed. The information obtained in such studies should be used to time biological sampling to minimize the impact of recent alcohol withdrawal on putative biological trait variables in patients with alcoholism.

Based on studies on the duration of biochemical effects of antidepressant withdrawal in humans, we have elected to start detailed investigations on neurotransmitter metabolism in alcoholics no sooner than after 21 days of abstinence.

ENVIRONMENTAL VARIABLES

Seasons have been known to affect functioning of the serotonergic neurones in the central nervous system. Our collaborative studies with investigators at the National Institute of Mental Health have shown that healthy volunteers have lowest CSF 5-HIAA concentrations in late winter and early spring.[19] Because the CSF 5-HIAA concentration varies seasonally by 40% in volunteers, patients and controls have to be carefully matched for the season of sampling in addition to a host of demographic variables, such as age, sex, and body build.[20]

Probably due to differences in stress and physical activity prior to sampling, healthy volunteers who have their lumbar punctures as either in or outpatients have significantly different CSF 5-HIAA concentrations from each other.[21] Thus, any valid comparisons across diagnostic groups require matching for in and outpatient status.

ALCOHOLISM AND SEROTONIN

Because diagnostic subgrouping of alcoholics has been controversial and many variables influencing CSF 5-HIAA concentration have been unknown, some differences in findings between various groups of investigators are to be expected. Therefore, it is remarkable that certain relatively consistent findings have emerged. Several groups have reported alcoholics, who have been abstinent for two to four weeks, to have lower CSF 5-HIAA concentrations than various control populations,[17,18,22] although there are negative reports as well.[23]

A relatively low CSF 5-HIAA concentration may be a trait variable in Type II alcoholics.[24] Our own studies have associated a low CSF 5-HIAA particularly with disorders of impulse control in criminal populations with alcoholism,[25,26] Furthermore, a low mean CSF

5-HIAA concentration has also been found in depressed patients with alcoholic relatives compared to depressed patients without alcoholic relatives.[27] Thus, a low CSF 5-HIAA may even be a familial trait.

ALCOHOLISM AND NOREPINEPHRINE

Another area of agreement in the neurotransmitter-alcoholism literature concerns noradrenergic overactivity during alcohol withdrawal. Both central and peripheral noradrenergic overactivity are associated with symptoms of alcohol withdrawal.[28-30] Furthermore, both the severity and duration of withdrawal symptoms correlate strongly with the degree of noradrenergic overactivity.[31] The cause of the excessive noradrenergic activity during alcohol withdrawal is somewhat unclear, but recent studies are suggestive of alcohol-induced changes in GABA (Paul S, Suszdak P, Karanian J, unpublished) and epinephrine[32] systems in the brain contributing to the overactivity. Also, indices of low noradrenergic activity have been reported in long term abstinent alcoholics.[33]

IMPLICATIONS OF THE FINDINGS

Recent explosive accumulation of knowledge in neurosciences in general and in neuropharmacology in particular will soon provide new, highly specific medications for the clinicians armamentarium. Therefore, knowledge concerning well defined neurochemical changes in relatively homogenous subgroups of alcoholics, and during various phases of the illness, is important for the provision of a scientific rationale for specific prevention and treatment strategies for alcoholism and its complications.

REFERENCES

1. Robins LN, Helzer JE, Weissman MM, Orvaschel H, Gruenberg E, Burke JP, Regier DA. Lifetime prevalence of specific psychiatric disorders in three sites. Arch Gen Psychiatry 1984; 41:949-58.
2. American Psychiatric Association: Diagnostic and Statistical Manual for Mental Disorders, 3rd edition, Washington, DC, 1980.

3. Schuckit M, Pitts FN, Reich T, King LJ, Winokur G. Alcoholism 1. Two types of alcoholism in women. Arch Gen Psychiatry 1969; 20:301-6.

4. Winokur G, Rimmer J, Reich T. Alcoholism IV. Is there more than one type of alcoholism. Brit J Psychiatry 1971; 118:525-31.

5. Hesselbrock MN. Women alcoholics: a comparison of the natural history of alcoholism between men and women. Document #58829. Rockville, MD: The National Clearinghouse for Alcohol Information, 1979.

6. Cadoret RJ, Gath A. Inheritance of alcoholism in adoptees. Brit J Psychiatry 1978; 132:252-8.

7. Goodwin DW, Schulsinger F, Moller N, Hermansen L, Winokur G, Guze SB. Drinking problems in adopted and non-adopted sons of alcoholics. Arch Gen Psychiatry 1974; 31:164-9.

8. Bohman M. Some genetic aspects of alcoholism and criminality: A population of adoptees. Arch Gen Psychiatry 1978; 35:269-76.

9. Cloninger CR, Bohman M, Sigvardsson S. Inheritance of alcohol abuse: Cross-fostering analysis of alcoholic men. Arch Gen Psychiatry 1981; 38:861-8.

10. Tarter RE, McBride H, Buonpane N, Schneider DU. Differentiation of alcoholics. Arch Gen Psychiatry 1977; 34:761-8.

11. Gittelman-Klein R, Mannuzza S, Shenker R, Bonagura N. Hyperactive children almost grown up. Arch Gen Psychiatry 1985; 42:937-47.

12. Weiss G, Torkenberg-Hechtman L. Hyperactive children grown up. New York: The Guilford Press, 1986.

13. Linnoila M, Martin PR. Benzodiazepines and alcoholism. In: Trimble MR, ed. Benzodiazepines divided. London: John Wiley and Sons Ltd, 1983:291-308.

14. Asberg M, Nordstrom P, Traskman-Benz L. Biological factors in suicide. In: Roy A, ed. Suicide. Baltimore: Williams & Wilkins, 1986:47-71.

15. Paykel E. Contribution of life events to causation of psychiatric illness. Psychol Med 1978; 8:245-53.

16. Roy A, Pickar D, Linnoila M, Doran AR, Paul SM. Cerebrospinal fluid monoamine and monoamine metabolite levels and the dexamethasone suppression test in depression. Arch Gen Psychiatry 1986; 43:356-60.

17. Banki CM. Factors influencing monoamine metabolites and tryptophan in patients with alcohol dependence. J Neural Transmission 1981; 50:89-101.

18. Borg S, Kvande H, Liljeberg P, Mossberg D, Valverius P. 5-hydroxyindoleacetic acid in cerebrospinal fluid in alcoholic patients under different conditions. Alcohol 1985; 2:415-8.

19. Brewerton TD, Berrettini WH, Nurnberger JI, Linnoila M. An analysis of seasonal fluctuations of CSF monoamine metabolites and neuropeptides in normal controls: findings with 5-HIAA and HVA. Psychiatry Res 1988; 23:257-65.

20. Agren H. Biological markers in major depressive disorders. A clinical and multivariate study. Uppsala, Acta Universitatis Upsaliensis 1981:405.

21. Guthrie SK, Berrettini WH, Rubinow DR, Nurnberger JI, Bartko JJ, Linnoila M. Different neurotransmitter metabolite concentrations in CSF samples

24 ALCOHOL RESEARCH FROM BENCH TO BEDSIDE

from inpatient and outpatient normal volunteers. Acta Psychiatr Scand 1986; 73:315-21.

22. Ballenger J, Goodwin F, Major L, Brown G. Alcohol and central serotonin metabolism in man. Arch Gen Psychiatry 1979; 36:224-7.

23. Takahasi S, Yamane H, Kondo H, Tani N, Kato N. CSF monoamine metabolites in alcoholism: a comparative study with depression. Folia Psychiatr Neurol Jap 1974; 28:43754.

24. Roy A, Virkkunen M, Linnoila M. Reduced central serotonin turnover in a subgroup of alcoholics? Progr Neuropsychopharmacol Biol Psychiatry 1987; 11:173-7.

25. Linnoila M, Virkkunen M, Scheinin M, Nuutila A, Rimon R, Goodwin FK. Low cerebrospinal fluid 5-hydroxyindoleacetic acid concentration differentiates impulsive from nonimpulsive violent behavior. Life Sci 1983; 33:2609-14.

26. Virkkunen M, Nuutila A, Goodwin FK, Linnoila M. Cerebrospinal fluid monoamine metabolite levels in male arsonist. Arch Gen Psychiatry 1987; 44:241-7.

27. Rosenthal N, Davenport Y, Cowdry R, Webster M, Goodwin F. Monoamine metabolites in cerebrospinal fluid of depressive subgroups. Psychiatry Res 1980; 2:113-9.

28. Borg S, Kvande H, Mossberg D, Valverius P, Sedvall G. Central nervous system noradrenaline metabolism and alcohol consumption in man. Pharmacol Biochem Behav 1983; 8, suppl 1:375-8.

29. Borg S, Liljeberg P, Mossberg D. Clinical studies on central noradrenergic activity in alcohol abusing patients. Acta Psychiatr Scand 1986; suppl 327:43-60.

30. Hawley RJ, Major LF, Schulman EA, Lake R. CSF levels of norepinephrine during alcohol withdrawal. Arch Neurol 1981; 38:289-92.

31. Hawley RJ, Major LF, Schulman EA, Linnoila M. Cerebrospinal fluid MHPG and NE in alcohol withdrawal: correlations with clinical signs. Arch Gen Psychiatry 1985; 42:1056-62.

32. Mefford. I, Karanian J, Ota M, Linnoila M. Depletion of hypothalamic epinephrine in rat brain during ethanol intoxication and withdrawal. Alcoholism, in press.

33. Borg S, Kvande H, Mossberg D, Sedvall G. Central nervous noradrenergic metabolism in alcoholics during long-term abstinence. Alcohol and Alcoholism 1983; 18:321-3.

The Aminopyrine Breath Test for the Evaluation of Liver Function in Alcoholic Patients: Drug Pharmacokinetics and Environmental Factors

Elizabeth A. Lane, PhD

SUMMARY. Drug pharmacokinetics and environmental factors contribute to the selection of an ideal drug substrate for the determination of liver function via the carbon dioxide breath test. An ideal drug should be rapidly absorbed, and have an hepatic extraction ratio between 0.2 and 0.5. Its metabolism should not be induced by ethanol or be affected by cigarette smoking. The relative promise of caffeine and methacetin are compared to aminopyrine.

The aminopyrine breath test has been advocated as a means of evaluation of liver function over the past ten years. It depends upon measurement of the excretion rate of a metabolite of aminopyrine after a single oral dose. Either the rate of excretion of the metabolite (carbon dioxide) at some specified time after the dose, or the cumulative fraction of the dose excreted as carbon dioxide up to some time (e.g., 2 hours) is usually measured. The carbon atom of the carbon dioxide from aminopyrine is labeled with an identifiable isotope of carbon (^{13}C or ^{14}C), which is incorporated into an aminopyrine methyl group, that is removed by oxidative metabolism in the

Elizabeth A. Lane is affiliated with the Section of Clinical Biochemical and Pharmacology, Laboratory of Clinical Studies, Division of Intramural Clinical and Biological Research, National Institute on Alcohol Abuse and Alcoholism, NIH Clinical Center, Bldg. 10, Rm. 3C213, Bethesda, MD 20892.

liver. So, the rate of hepatic metabolism of aminopyrine has become the basis of measurement of the functional capacity of the liver. The underlying assumption of the test is that the demethylation of aminopyrine is the rate-limiting step in the appearance of labeled CO_2 in expired breath.

The aminopyrine breath test was first described by Lauterburg and Bircher[1] in 1973. Soon afterwards, Hepner and Vesell[2] and Lauterburg and Bircher[3] demonstrated in man and rat, respectively, that states of increased or decreased aminopyrine plasma clearance resulted in a corresponding increase or decrease in the aminopyrine breath test result. Hepner and Vesell[2] reported that the aminopyrine breath test result was lower in portal cirrhosis patients than in healthy volunteers and that known inhibitors and inducers of aminopyrine metabolism decreased and increased the breath test result, respectively. In addition, the excretion of $^{14}CO_2$ in 12 hours[2] and in 2 hours,[4] was linearly related to the plasma clearance of aminopyrine, thereby, lending support to the assumption that the demethylation of aminopyrine is the rate-limiting step in the rate of excretion of the CO_2.

Since this initial work, a number of investigators have compared the aminopyrine breath test to other measures of liver function as a means of diagnosing alcoholic liver disease of various severity. Most agree that the aminopyrine breath test clearly separates patients with hepatic cirrhosis from other patients.[5,6,7,8,9] In such patients the aminopyrine breath test results were significantly correlated with sulphobromophthalein retention,[5,6] galactose elimination,[6] prothrombin time,[9] and postprandial bile acids,[7] and sometimes correlated with serum albumin.[5,9] However, there is some disagreement regarding the usefulness of the aminopyrine breath test in the detection of alcoholic liver disease.[10,11] On the one hand, Galizzi et al.[10] found that the aminopyrine breath test was no better than SGOT or 2 hour postprandial bile acids for diagnosis of minimal alcoholic liver disease described as fatty liver by biopsy. On the other hand, Saunders et al.[11] showed that the aminopyrine breath test could separate alcoholics with compensated cirrhosis when it was carried out within 48 hours of admission for detoxification. After 7-10 days of abstinence the aminopyrine breath test was within the normal range in half of those patients. However, in alcoholics with fatty changes to the liver or with portal fibrosis the results were very variable and distributed across the normal range.

The results of Saunders et al.[11] illustrate one of the effects of alcohol abuse upon aminopyrine clearance that tends to confound the use of this test in early diagnosis of alcoholic liver disease. Namely, within 48 hours of admission the aminopyrine breath test results in alcoholic patients with normal liver histology were significantly greater than in a control group, indicating that alcohol can increase aminopyrine clearance, probably by induction of enzymes. This tendency of alcohol abuse to increase aminopyrine clearance camouflages any tendency of fatty changes or fibrosis to decrease it, thereby resulting in apparently normal aminopyrine breath test results in these patients.

As a result of variability in opinion regarding the usefulness of the aminopyrine breath test as a liver function test, several factors that might influence the outcome of the test have been considered. These include, (1) factors having to do with the drug used, i.e., the pharmacokinetic characteristics of aminopyrine compared to the pharmacokinetics of other drugs that have been proposed for this test (caffeine,[12,13,14] phenacetin,[15,16] methacetin,[17,18] diazepam[19]); and (2) the interaction of environmental factors or patient habits with drug elimination.

DRUG PHARMACOKINETICS AND THE AMINOPYRINE BREATH TEST

The effect of pharmacokinetic parameters, including hepatic extraction ratio, fraction metabolised by demethylation, volume of distribution, half-life and absorption rate constant, upon the outcome of a breath test have been modeled and described in detail elsewhere.[20] In brief, although all of these factors can affect the shape of the expired CO_2 curve, the most important one when determining variability in liver function via the CO_2 breath test is hepatic extraction ratio (E), i.e., the fraction of the oral dose that is metabolized during its first pass through the liver. The fraction of the dose expired as CO_2 within 2 hours of the dose is curvilinearly related to plasma clearance. Drugs having high extraction ratios are predicted to be insensitive probes of liver function via the CO_2 breath test.

This is because the fraction of the dose eliminated as CO_2 in 2 hours barely changes for a large change in plasma clearance. However for drugs having an extraction ratio below 0.5 this expression of the breath test result is reasonably sensitive to variability in drug clearance and, therefore, to variability in liver function. For such lower extraction ratio drugs this relationship could be approximated by a straight line similar to the linear correlation reported by other investigators.[2,4,13] These simulations led to the conclusion that a drug suitable for determination of liver function via the breath test should have an extraction ratio 0.2 to 0.5. The extraction ratios of drugs suggested for use in this test extend over most of the possible range of extraction ratios (0 to 1.0) but the extraction ratio of aminopyrine, the drug used for the development of this method, is within this favorable range: 0.2. In comparison, methacetin and phenacetin E = 0.8 to 1.0; caffeine C = 0.1-0.2; diazepam E < 0.1.

ENVIRONMENTAL FACTORS AND THE AMINOPYRINE BREATH TEST

Drug clearance is determined by genetic and environmental factors. The effects of certain environmental factors may be important in the application of the breath test depending upon the substrate used. It is known that cigarette smoking and certain anticonvulsant drugs as well as ethanol are inducers of some enzymes responsible for the metabolism of the drugs used in the breath test (see Table 1).

The effect of cigarette smoking or treatment with carbamazepine and phenytoin on the breath test results from caffeine and methacetin are illustrated in Figures 1 and 2, respectively. Both factors increased the fraction of the dose excreted as CO_2 in two hours, compared with a healthy control subject, but the increase is more pronounced for the lower extraction ratio drug (caffeine) than for the high extraction ration drug (methacetin). Similarly, the increased clearance of aminopyrine in an alcoholic patient abstinent for 24 hours, compared with a smoker and nonsmoker volunteers is illustrated in Figure 3. Since more than half of the alcoholic patients seen at many institutions are cigarette smokers, any effect of cigarette smoking upon drug disposition is a potentially confounding factor in the interpretation of a caffeine or methacetin breath test used to evaluate liver function in an alcoholic patient.

TABLE 1. Induction of metabolism of CO_2 breath test substrates by environmental factors and drug treatments.

	CIGARETTES	PHENOBARBITAL	PHENYTOIN	ETHANOL
AMINOPYRINE	---[21]	+[19,21]	+[19]	+[11]
CAFFEINE	+[13]	---[14]		---[22]
METHACETIN	? +[21]	? +[21,23]		
DIAZEPAM		+[19]	+[19]	? +[24,25]

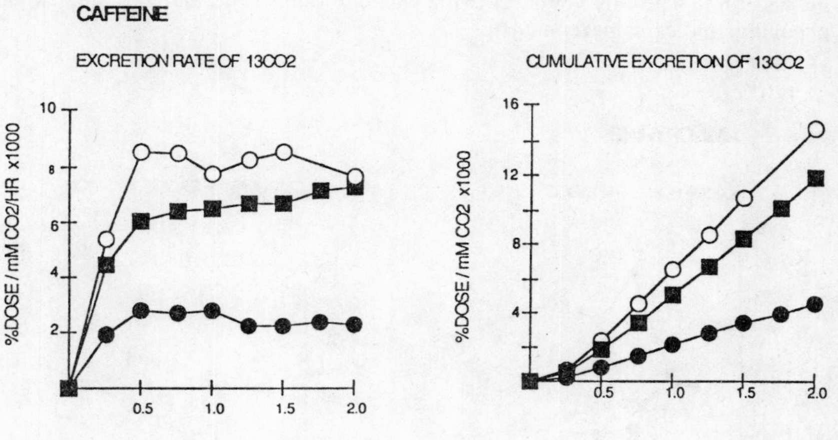

CAFFEINE

EXCRETION RATE OF 13CO2

CUMULATIVE EXCRETION OF 13CO2

FIGURE 1. Excretion rate and cumulative excretion of $^{13}CO_2$ after a single dose of caffeine to a healthy volunteer [●], a cigarette smoker [o], and a patient taking phenytoin and carbamazepine [■].

These data demonstrate the importance of taking account of the pharmacokinetics of a drug and the interaction of various environmental factors with the clearance of the drug when it is evaluated as probe for alcoholic liver disease via the carbon dioxide breath test. An ideal drug should have an extraction ratio less than 0.5 and its

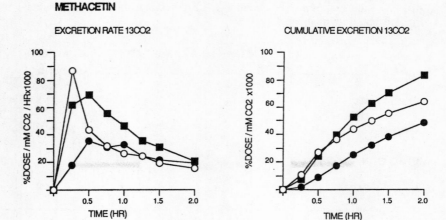

FIGURE 2. Excretion rate and cumulative excretion of $^{13}CO_2$ after a single dose of methacetin to a healthy volunteer [●], a cigarette smoker [o], and a patient taking phenytoin and carbamazepine [■].

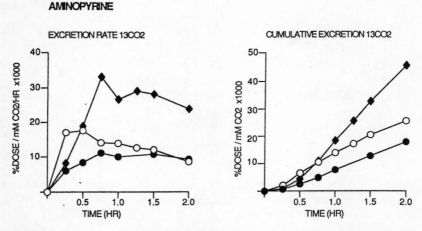

FIGURE 3. Excretion rate and cumulative excretion of $^{13}CO_2$ after a single dose of aminopyrine to a healthy volunteer [●], a cigarette smoker [o], and an alcoholic patient 24 hours after his last drink [◆].

metabolism should not be induced by cigarette smoking or alcohol. In addition it is desirable that the test drug should have no pharmacological action. None of the four compounds reviewed here is an ideal probe by these criteria and each should be used with an awareness of its limitations. That is, aminopyrine will detect compensated cirrhosis but not fatty changes or fibrosis of the liver; caffeine may be a more sensitive probe of early alcoholic liver disease in nonsmoking patients, but these are a minority. Information regarding the usefulness of methacetin is more limited. It should be a less sensitive probe than caffeine because of its high extraction ratio; it suffers similar limitations as caffeine if its clearance is induced by cigarette smoking as seems likely (Figure 2 and Table 1); and whether its clearance is induced by alcohol is unknown at this time.

REFERENCES

1. Lauterburg BH, Bircher J. Hepatic microsomal drug metabolizing capacity measured in vivo by breath analysis. Gastroenterology 1973; 65:556.

2. Hepner GW, Vesell ES. Assessment of aminopyrine metabolism in man by breath analysis after oral administration of ^{14}C-aminopyrine. Effects of phenobarbital, disulfiram and portal cirrhosis. N Engl J Med 1974; 291:1384-1388.

3. Lauterburg BH, Bircher J. Expiratory measurement of maximal aminopyrine demethylation *in vivo*: Effect of phenobarbital, partial hepatectomy, portacaval shunt and bile duct ligation in the rat. J Pharmacol Exp Ther 1976; 196:501-509.

4. Hepner GW, Vesell ES. Aminopyrine disposition: Studies on breath, saliva, and urine of normal subjects and patients with liver disease. Clin Pharmacol Ther 1976; 20:654-660.

5. Hepner GW, Vesell ES. Quantitative assessment of hepatic function by breath analysis after oral administration of [^{14}C]aminopyrine. Ann Intern Med 1975; 83:632-638.

6. Bircher J, Kupfer A, Gikalov I, Preisig R. Aminopyrine demethylation measured by breath analysis in cirrhosis. Clin Pharmacol Ther 1976; 20:484-492.

7. Galizzi J, Long RG, Billing BH, Sherlock S. Assessment of the (^{14}C)aminopyrine breath test in liver disease. Gut 1978; 19:40-45.

8. Noordhoek J, Dees J, Savenije-Chapel EM, Wilson JHP. Output of ^{14}CO$_2$ in breath after oral administration of (^{14}C-methyl)aminopyrine in hepatitis, cirrhosis and hepatic bilharziasis: Its relationship to aminopyrine pharmacokinetics. Europ J clin Pharmacol 1978; 13:223-229.

9. Carlisle R, Galambos JT, Warren WD. The relationship between conventional liver tests, quantitative function tests and histopathology in cirrhosis. Dig Dis Sci 1979; 24:358-362.

10. Galizzi J, Morgan MY, Chitranukroh A, Sherlock S. The detection of

minimal alcoholic liver disease by three methods. Scand J Gastroenterol 1978; 13:827-831.

11. Saunders JB, Lewis KO, Paton A. Early diagnosis of alcoholic cirrhosis by the aminopyrine breath test. Gastroenterology 1980; 79:112-114.

12. Renner E, Wietholtz H, Huguenin P, Arnaud MJ, Preisig R. Caffeine: A model compound for measuring liver function. Hepatology 1984; 4:38-46.

13. Kotake AN, Schoeller DA, Lambert GH, Baker AL, Schaffer DD, Josephs H. The caffeine CO_2 breath test: Dose response and route of N-demethylation in smokers and nonsmokers. Clin Pharamcol Ther 1982; 32:261-269.

14. Wietholtz H, Voegelin M, Arnaud MJ, Bircher J, Preisig R. Assessment of the cytochrome P-448 dependent liver enzyme system by a caffeine breath test. Eur J clin Pharmacol 1981; 21:53-59.

15. Breen KJ, Bury RW, Calder IV, Desmond PV, Peters M, Mashford ML. A [14C]phenacetin breath test to measure hepatic function in man. Hepatology 1984; 4:47-52.

16. Schoeller DA, Kotake AN, Lambert GH, Krager PS, Baker AL. Comparison of the phenacetin and aminopyrine breath tests: Effect of liver disease, inducers and cobaltous chloride. Hepatology 1985; 5:276-281.

17. Fahl J, Wong W, Klein PD, Watkins JB. $^{13}CO_2$ methacetin breath test for hepatic function-A noninvasive approach. Hepatology 1984; 4:1094.

18. Fahl J, Kaplan R, Antonow D, Wong W, Klein PD, Soloway R, Watkins JB. $^{13}CO_2$ methacetin breath test: A comparative analysis. Hepatology 1984; 4:1094.

19. Hepner GW, Vesell ES, Lipton A, Harvey HA, Wilkinson GR, Schenker S. Disposition of aminopyrine, diazepam and indocyanine green in patients with liver disease or an anticonvulsant therapy: Diazepam breath test and correlation in drug elimination. J Lab Clin Med 1977; 90:440-456.

20. Lane EA, Parashos I. Drug pharmacokinetics and the carbon dioxide breath test. J Pharmacokin Biopharm 1986; 14:29-49.

21. Schneider JF, Schoeller DA, Schreider BD, Kotake AN, Hachey DL, Klein PD. Use óf ^{13}C-phenacetin and ^{13}C-methacetin for the detection of alterations in hepatic drug metabolism. In: Klein ER, Klein PD, ed. Stable isotopes: proceedings of the third international conference. New York: Academic Press, 1979:507-516.

22. Mitchell MC, Hoyumpa AM, Schenker S, Patwardhan PV. Differential effects of chronic ethanol feeding on cytochrome P-448 and P-450-mediated drug metabolism in the rat. Biochem Pharmacol 1982; 31:695-699.

23. Thornhill DP, Steffen C, Netter KJ. A kinetic evaluation of $^{14}CO_2$ in expired air after ^{14}C-methacetin administration in rats, used for the *in vivo* study of the metabolism of drugs. Eur J Drug Metab and Pharmacokin 1984; 9:161-168.

24. Pond SM, Phillips M, Benowitz NI, Galinsky RE, Tong TG, Becker CE. Diazepam kinetics in acute alcohol withdrawal. Clin Pharmacol Ther 1979; 25:832-836.

25. Sellers EM, Sandor P, Giles HG, Khouw V, Greenblatt DJ. Diazepam pharmacokinetics after intravenous administration in alcohol withdrawal. Br J Clin Pharmacol 1983; 15:125-127.

The Measurement of D,L-2,3-Butanediol in Controls and Patients with Alcoholic Cirrhosis

J. P. Casazza, PhD
J. Freitas, MD
D. Stambuk, MD
M. Y. Morgan, MD
R. L. Veech, MD, DPhil

SUMMARY. Plasma D,L-2,3-butanediol was measured in 53 controls and 50 patients with alcoholic cirrhosis, none of whom had measurable amounts of blood ethanol. Thirteen of 50 samples from patients with alcoholic cirrhosis had measurable D,L-2,3-butanediol. (range < 5-154 uM). In one patient with alcoholic cirrhosis who had been abstinent from ethanol for over 5 years plasma levels of D,L-2,3-butanediol ranged between 154 and 211 uM over a one-year period. Only one of the 53 control subjects had detectable levels of D,L-2,3-butanediol. Although it has previously been reported that 2,3-butanediol is present in alcoholics consuming distilled spirits (Rutstein et al. (1983) Lancet ii, 534), this is the first report of the persistent presence of these compounds in alcoholics in the absence of ethanol. Clearly in abstinent alcoholics the presence of 2,3-butanediol is not due to the ingestion of undistilled spirits nor is it likely to arise directly from the metabolic products of ethanol. The presence of D,L-2,3-butanediol in patients with alcoholic cirrhosis and its absence in control subjects suggests that this compound may be a marker of some forms for alcoholism.

J. P. Casazza and R. L. Veech are affiliated with the Laboratory of Metabolism and Molecular Biology, National Institute on Alcohol Abuse and Alcoholism, 12501 Washington Avenue, Rockville, MD 20852. J. Freitas, D. Stambuk, and M. Y. Morgan are affiliated with the Royal Free Hospital, Academic Department of Medicine, London, England.

Requests for reprints should be addressed to J. P. Casazza.

Plasma D,L-2,3-butanediol was measured by the method of Needham et al.[1] in 53 controls and 50 patients with biopsy-proven alcoholic cirrhosis, none of whom had measurable amounts of blood ethanol. Thirteen of 50 samples from patients with alcoholic cirrhosis had measurable D,L-2,3-butanediol (range < 5-154 uM). In one patient with alcoholic cirrhosis who had been abstinent from ethanol for over 5 years plasma levels of D,L-2,3-butanediol ranged between 154 and 211 uM over a one-year period. Only one of the 53 control subjects had detectable levels of D,L-2,3-butanediol (range < 5-5 uM). There was no correlation between serum alkaline phosphatase activity, SGOT activity, serum albumin and serum bilirubin and the incidence of D,L-2,3-butanediol. Nor was there any difference in the incidence of D,L-2,3-butanediol in patients that were ethanol abstinent for a period of more than a week (38 patients) and those that were not (12 patients).

The presence of 2,3-butanediol has previously been reported in alcoholics when blood ethanol was present. Rutstein et al.[2] measured 2,3-butanediol in alcoholics admitted to a detoxification ward who had been drinking only distilled spirits. In samples drawn from alcoholics at the time of admission in which blood ethanol was measurable 15 of 19 samples contained measurable, 2,3-butanediol (range < 5-101 uM). Although not reported by Rutstein et al.[2] 8 of these 19 samples contained measurable D,L-2,3-butanediol (range < 5-34 uM). In samples drawn from these same alcoholics 36 hours after admission only 4 of 18 samples contained 2,3-butanediol (range < 5-36 uM). All four of these samples contained D,L-2,3-butanediol. Only one of 22 control subjects contained measurable 2,3-butanediol in either the presence or absence of ethanol. This difference in the incidence and concentration of 2,3-butanediol in alcoholics in the presence and absence of measurable blood ethanol led Rutstein et al.[2] to postulate that 2,3-butanediol production in alcoholics was the result of an aberrant pathway of ethanol metabolism in alcoholics. The presence of D,L-2,3-butanediol in alcohol abstinent patients with alcoholic cirrhosis indicates that in these samples 2,3-butanediol is not a by-product of ethanol metabolism. Nonetheless the presence of 2,3-butanediol at an increased frequency in alcoholics when consuming ethanol than in its absence suggests that ethanol plays some role in the production of 2,3-butanediol in alcoholics even if it is not the direct metabolic product of ethanol. These data suggest that in future studies the presence of alcoholic cirrhosis must be taken into consideration when studying the incidence of diols in alcoholics.

REFERENCES

1. Needham LL, Hill RH, Orti DL, Felver ME, Liddle JA. Electron capture, capillary column gas chromatographic determination of low molecular weight diols in serum. J. Chromatogr. 1982; 233:9-17.
2. Rutstein DD, Veech RL, Nickerson RJ, Felver ME, Vernon AA, Needham LL, Kishore P, and Thacker SB. 2,3-Butanediol: An unusual metabolite in the serum of severely alcoholic men during acute intoxication. Lancet. 1983; ii:534-537.

Circadian Rhythms of Cortisol During Alcohol Withdrawal

Debra Risher-Flowers, MD, PhD
Bryon Adinoff, MD
Bernard Ravitz, MD
George H. A. Bone, MD
Peter R. Martin, MD
David Nutt, MD, PhD
Markku Linnoila, MD, PhD

SUMMARY. The authors have investigated the function of the hypothalamic-pituitary-adrenocortical (HPA) axis during and after withdrawal from alcohol. 24 hour rhythms of cortisol were abnormal in that elevated levels were seen throughout the day in patients with moderate to severe, but not mild, withdrawal. This abnormality of circadian secretion of cortisol, which is similar to that seen in Cushing's syndrome and post-operative trauma, returned to normal after a period of one week of abstinence on their in-patient ward. Such excessive secretion of cortisol may explain some of the complications of chronic alcoholism.

Numerous hormonal changes have been associated with both the acute and chronic use of alcohol as well as the alcohol withdrawal syndrome.[1] Many of these alterations have been linked to abnormalities of the hypothalamic-pituitary-adrenal (HPA) axis.[2] The activation of this system results in increased levels of adrenocorticotropic hormone and cortisol. It is reported to be associated with the devel-

The authors are affiliated with the Laboratory of Clinical Studies, Division of Intramural Clinical and Biological Research, National Institute on Alcohol Abuse and Alcoholism, NIH Clinical Center, Bldg. 10, Rm. 3C103, Bethesda, MD 20892.

Reprint requests should be addressed to Debra Risher-Flowers.

opment of tolerance to alcohol, depressive and Cushing's-like syndromes, and the degree of severity of symptoms experienced during withdrawal from alcohol.

The intent of the present study was to determine the alterations in HPA axis function during the symptomatic phase of acute withdrawal from alcohol and following its resolution. Although disturbances in the circadian pattern of corticosteroid concentrations have been reported during the alcohol withdrawal syndrome in both human,[3,5] and animal[4] studies, these changes have not been well described. To further elucidate such changes, we measured plasma levels of cortisol every thirty minutes for 24 hours on the first, third, and seventh day following abstinence in subjects with alcohol dependence.

All subjects were studied on the NIAAA inpatient research unit of the Clinical Center located at the National Institutes of Health. Four male subjects (42 ± 4.3 years) had been previously evaluated for adherence to criteria for alcohol dependence according to the Diagnostic and Statistical Manual of Mental Disorders, third edition (DSM III) and absence of additional psychopathology, including other substance use disorders, or a history of neurologic or neuroendocrine dysfunction. At the time of admission, subjects had no significant medical disorders as documented by physical examination or laboratory findings. Patients were admitted at approximately 9 a.m. for participation in studies. Measures of blood alcohol concentrations (BACs) and objective ratings of the severity of alcohol withdrawal using the Clinical Institute Withdrawal Assessment-Alcohol (CIWA-A) scale were obtained hourly. Signs and symptoms of withdrawal were managed by supportive measures. Beginning at 5 p.m. on the day of admission, plasma cortisol levels were obtained at half hour intervals for a total of twenty-four hours (DAY 1). Subsequent 24-hour cortisol measurements were made beginning twenty-four hours (DAY 3) and one week (DAY 7) later. Additionally, hourly cortisol levels were obtained over a twenty-four hour period in six male subjects (53.8 ± 8.2 years) who were in good health and free of drugs, and served as controls.

The four patients in this study were admitted with BACs ranging up to 180 mg%. All BACs had declined to undetectable levels by 9 p.m. on Day 1 of the study. Three patients were rated as having moderate withdrawal as indicated by symptoms of marked autonomic hyperactivity, significant psychologic distress, and psychosensory distortions (peak CIWA-A = 20-25). Peak CIWA-A scores characteristically occurred when BACs became undetectable and were sustained for three to five hours before beginning a gradual decline over the subsequent twelve to twenty-four hours. All three patients rated as experiencing moderate withdrawal exhibited elevated cortisol levels throughout DAY 1 (mean SD = 16.0 ± 4.4 ug/dl) with return to control levels (10.8 ± 0.5 ug/dl) by DAY 7 (9.2 ± 1.04 ug/dl) (Figure 1). In addition to cortisol elevations on DAY 1, two of these patients exhibited an absence of diurnal rhythmicity for cortisol secretion exhibited by sustained elevations of cortisol throughout the first 24 hours. The fourth patient experienced only mild withdrawal symptoms as reflected in a peak CIWA-A score of 9. His levels and rhythms of cortisol secretion were similar to the control values on all three test days.

These preliminary findings demonstrate a greater than 40% increase in cortisol levels on DAY 1 versus DAY 7 and a disturbance of circadian rhythmicity in patients experiencing moderate to severe withdrawal. These changes are similar in magnitude to the values observed in patients with severe malnutrition, post-operative trauma or Cushings syndrome and indicate a significant activation of the HPA axis. The reversal of cortisol elevations and restoration of diurnal rhythm by DAY 7 may suggest that adrenal function is initially maximally stimulated, or that there is an activation of a preexisting abnormality of circadian rhythm or a combination of these two factors occurring during acute withdrawal from alcohol. These alterations may explain certain signs and symptoms of the alcohol withdrawal syndrome such as weakness, fatigue, mental confusion, and depression. Furthermore, repeated bouts of elevated cortisol during successive withdrawal episodes may result in hippocampal damage and development of an organic brain syndrome.

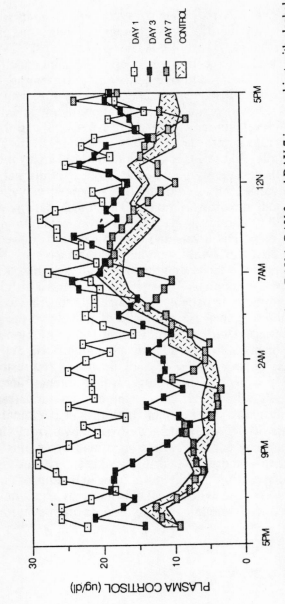

TOTAL PLASMA CORTISOL ON DAY 1, DAY 3 AND DAY 7 DURING ALCOHOL WITHDRAWAL

FIGURE 1. Cortisol levels obtained at half-hour intervals on DAY 1, DAY 3, and DAY 7 in one subject with alcohol dependence following abstinence from alcohol and the subsequent development of a moderately severe alcohol withdrawal syndrome. BAC was 180 mg% and CIWA-A 10 on admission. Peak withdrawal symptomatology occurred at 7pm on DAY 1 (CIWA-A = 25). DAY 1 mean cortisol values reveal a 300 percent elevation over DAY 7 levels in this patient and also demonstrate an absence of circadian rhythm. Comparison is also made to circadian rhythmicity of cortisol in six healthy male subjects.

40

NOTES

1. Cicero, TJ. Neuroendocrinological effects of alcohol. Ann Rev Med. 1981; 32:123-142.

2. Mendelson, JH, and Stein, S. Serum cortisol levels in alcoholics and nonalcoholic subjects during experimentally induced ethanol intoxication. Psychosomatic Medicine. 1966, 28:616-26.

3. Noth, RH, and Walter, RM. The effects of alcohol on the endocrine system. Medical Clinics of North America. 1984, 68:133-46.

4. Tabakoff, B, Jaffe, RC, and Ritzmann, RF. Corticosterone concentrations in mice during ethanol drinking and withdrawal. J Pharm Pharmacol. 1978, 30:371-74.

5. Valimaki, M, Pelkonen, R, Harkonen, M, and Ylikahri, R. Hormonal changes in noncirrhotic male alcoholics during ethanol withdrawal. Alcohol and Alcoholism. 1984, 19:235-42.

Alpha-2-Adrenoceptor Function in Alcoholics

David J. Nutt, MD, PhD
Paul Glue, MD

SUMMARY. Alpha-2-adrenoceptor function has been assessed using the iv clonidine challenge test. During withdrawal clonidine effects on blood pressure, sedation and body temperature were blunted compared with the abstinent state and healthy controls. In contrast the growth hormone response was blunted in both the withdrawing and abstinent alcoholics. These findings suggest that a deficit of alpha-2-inhibitory control is a feature of withdrawal and, in the case of the endocrine response, may persist for some time.

For many years it has been appreciated that alcohol interacts with brain monoamine systems.[1] The present article presents some recent work on ethanol-norepinephrine interactions in man. In particular we examine the possibility that dysfunction or subsensitivity of alpha-2-adrenoceptors might account for many of the phenomena of withdrawal.

It is now well established that overactivity of brain and peripheral norepinephrine systems occurs in alcohol withdrawal.[2] For instance many of the symptoms of withdrawal are those of sympathetic nervous system overactivity which may be mediated by increased firing of the locus coeruleus. Since central norepinephrine release may

The authors are affiliated with the Section of Clinical Science, Laboratory of Clinical Studies, Division of Intramural Clinical and Biological Research, National Institute on Alcohol Abuse and Alcoholism, NIH Clinical Center, Bldg. 10, Rm. 3B19, Bethesda, MD 20892. The clinical studies described were carried out in part with funding from the Wellcome Trust. Dr. Nutt is a Wellcome Senior Fellow in Clinical Science.

Reprint requests should be addressed to Dr. Nutt.

be increased by reductions of alpha-2-adrenoceptor input (see 3) we investigated the sensitivity of this receptor in alcoholics during withdrawal using the alpha-2-adrenoceptor agonist clonidine. This drug has the advantage of reducing withdrawal symptoms[4] and so it is an ethically and clinically acceptable probe. To avoid possible pharmacokinetic problems we used an intravenous infusion of clonidine (1.5 ug/kg) and monitored psychological and physiological variables for the next 90 min.

As expected from the earlier oral studies clonidine reduced withdrawal symptomatology as well as blood pressure, heart rate and plasma MHPG. However when compared with an age- and sex-matched normal control population the alcoholics showed a relative subsensitivity to the hypotensive and sedative effects of clonidine (Table 1), and these actions were not simply due to altered basal levels of these variables in alcoholics, since in essential hypertension the response to clonidine is exaggerated.[5] Furthermore in the alcoholics sedation was reduced despite them being more aroused (less sedated) at baseline.[6]

Body temperature is reduced by clonidine; however in the with-

Table 1.

Clonidine sensitivity in alcoholics during withdrawal and in abstinence compared with age- and sex-matched controls

Clonidine action	Withdrawal	Abstinence
hypotension	-	nc
bradycardia	nc	nc
hypothermia	-	nc
plasma MHPG decrease	+	?
growth hormone release	-	-
sedation	-	nc

+: increased, -: decreased, nc: no change. ?: not available.

drawing alcoholics this action was abolished and slight increase in temperature was observed over the course of the study (Table 1).

These results are compatible with reduced alpha-2-inhibitory control of the locus coeruleus in alcohol withdrawal, with the subsequent increase of norepinephrine output from the brain and periphery.

Another observation that emerges from this study is that there was a strong positive correlation between plasma levels of MHPG and the number of previous episodes of withdrawal for each alcoholic ($r = 0.92$, $p < 0.005$). This offers some pharmacological support for the suggestion that repeated episodes of withdrawal might sensitize (or kindle) the brain.[7] If this were to occur in the norepinephrine system it might make future withdrawal more likely or severe. These results need to be repeated, preferably with CSF measures of MHPG as well as norepinephrine, epinephrine and other metabolites, in order to exclude the possibility that peripheral metabolic factors might explain the observation.

We have also been able to perform clonidine testing in alcoholics that have been sober for 4-5 weeks in a treatment unit (see Table 1). In these patients the effects of clonidine on blood pressure and the heart rate were the same as in normal controls, and the baseline levels of these variables had returned to normal. The temperature reduction in response to clonidine was also apparent to a normal extent. In contrast the growth hormone responses were still blunted with only 2 out of 9 alcoholics showing a response. Whether a longer period of abstinence would allow full recovery of this endocrine response is not yet clear but it is interesting that in depression these responses may be blunted even in euthymic drug-free patients.[8]

This body of data suggests alpha-2-adrenoceptor dysfunction (subsensitivity) during alcohol withdrawal which, except for the growth hormone response, returns to normal after a period of abstinence. It is possible that this dysfunction is causally related to the appearance of withdrawal symptoms and signs. Possible explanations for these findings may be provided by the recent animal work on the interactions between ethanol and the endogenous alpha-2-adrenoceptor ligand epinephrine which has shown that chronic ethanol administration depletes brain epinephrine concentrations.[9] If epinephrine's main function is to act as an endogenous inhibitor of norepinephrine release then this deficiency could lead to excessive norepinephrine activity during withdrawal. However, our findings of subsensitive alpha-2-adrenoceptors might argue in favour of a change at the receptor/cell membrane level.

Additionally the persistent blunting of the growth hormone response to clonidine in the abstinent alcoholics may indicate a degree of chronic noradrenergic dysfunction which might potentially provide a state or trait marker in alcoholics.

REFERENCES

1. Nutt DJ, Glue P. Alcohol and monoamines. Br J Addiction 1986; 81: 327-38.

2. Hawley RJ, Major LF, Schulman EA, Linnoila M. Cerebrospinal 3-methoxy-4-hydroxyphenolglycol and norepinephrine levels in alcohol withdrawal. Arch Gen Psych 1985; 42:1056-62.

3. Cedarbaum JM, Aghajanian GK. Noradrenergic neurons of the locus coruleus: inhibition by epinephrine and activation by the alpha-2-antagonist piperoxane. Brain Res 1976; 112:413-19.

4. Bjorkquist SE. Clonidine in alcohol withdrawal. Acta Psych Scand 1975; 52:256-63.

5. Goldstein DS, Levinson PD, Zimlichman R, Pitterman A, Stull R, Keiser HR. Clonidine suppression testing in essential hypertension. Ann Int Med 1985; 103:42-8.

6. Glue P, Nutt DJ. Clonidine in alcohol withdrawal: a pilot study of differential symptom responses following i.v. clonidine. Alcohol Alcoholism 1987; 22:161-6.

7. Ballenger JC, Post RM. Kindling as a model for the alcohol withdrawal syndromes. Br J Psychiatry 1978; 133:1-14.

8. Siever L et al. Proc 42nd Biol Psych Meeting, Chicago, 1987.

9. Linnoila M, Mefford I, Nutt D, Adinoff B. Alcohol withdrawal and noradrenergic function. Ann Int Med 1987; 107:875-89.

Treatment of Alcoholic Organic Brain Syndrome with the Serotonin Reuptake Inhibitor Fluvoxamine: A Preliminary Study

J. M. Stapleton, PhD
M. J. Eckardt, PhD
P. Martin, MD
B. Adinoff, MD
L. Roehrich, BS
G. Bone, MD
D. Rubinow, MD
M. Linnoila, MD, PhD

SUMMARY. The chronic effects of fluvoxamine (200 mg per day for 4 weeks) were studied in ten alcoholic organic brain syndrome patients in a double-blind cross-over design. Complete neuropsychological evaluation was performed as well as measurement of neurochemical changes in CSF.

Fluvoxamine produced a small but significant improvement in memory performance. An analysis of fluvoxamine minus placebo difference scores showed a significant correlation between memory functioning and CSF 5HIAA levels. Alcohol amnestic syndrome patients who had the highest blood levels of fluvoxamine demonstrated the largest changes in CSF 5HIAA and improvement in memory performance under fluvoxamine. These findings implicate a role of serotonergic mechanisms in alcoholic organic brain syndrome and

All of the above authors, with the exception of D. Rubinow, are affiliated with the Section of Clinical Brain Research, Laboratory of Clinical Studies, Division of Intramural Clinical and Biological Research, National Institute on Alcohol Abuse and Alcoholism, NIH Clinical Center, Bldg. 10, Rm. 3C-218, Bethesda, MD 20892. D. Rubinow is affiliated with the National Institute of Mental Health.
Reprint requests should be sent to M. J. Eckardt.

47

suggest that with individual titration of the drug dose, fluvoxamine might be a clinically useful agent in the treatment of this syndrome.

Alcoholic organic brain syndrome includes a constellation of deficits, most prominently a profound impairment in episodic memory performance. It has been suggested that some of these deficits might be related to malfunction of the serotonin system.[1] This study was undertaken to determine whether manipulation of the serotonin system using fluvoxamine, a relatively specific serotonin reuptake inhibitor, could ameliorate any of these deficits.

METHODS

The effects of fluvoxamine (200 mg per day for 4 weeks) were studied in ten alcoholic organic brain syndrome patients in a double-blind cross-over design. Complete neuropsychological evaluation was performed as well as measurement of neurochemical changes in cerebrospinal fluid (CSF) obtained by lumbar puncture (LP). Patients were maintained on a low monoamine diet and no food or smoking was permitted after 12:01 a.m. on the day of the LP. Intravenous lines were inserted at least one hour prior to the procedure, and blood pressure and pulse were monitored at 5 min intervals. Immediately before the LP, 23 mls of blood were obtained via the intravenous line. All subjects were inpatients on the NIAAA treatment unit, and the LPs were performed in the patient's room between 8:30 and 9:30 a.m. Outside stimulation (e.g., television, radios, phone calls) was not permitted during the procedure. A total of 32 mls of CSF were obtained, aliquoted, and frozen at −70 C until assayed.

Neuropsychological assessment included the Wechsler Adult Intelligence Scale (WAIS),[2] the Wechsler Memory Scale (WMS),[3] the Halstead-Reitan Neuropsychological Battery,[4] and a test of episodic memory functioning.[5] Four patients were subsequently deleted from study — one due to refusal to consent to LP, one due to evidence of alcoholic liver disease, and two due to procedural problems. The remaining patients included five diagnosed as having alcohol amnestic syndrome and one with alcoholic dementia.

RESULTS

The characteristics of the patients are shown in Table 1.

Baseline levels of somatostatin in CSF were significantly correlated with the baseline measure of memory performance on the WMS memory quotient (MQ) (r = 0.80, p < .05), with neuropsychological impairment being associated with lower levels of somatostatin.

Table 2 shows the levels of several neurochemical and hormonal measures in CSF. There was a statistically significant decrease in CSF levels of 5-hydroxy-indole-acetic acid (5HIAA) as might be expected from a drug which blocks 5-hydroxytryptamine (5HT)

TABLE 1

	MEAN(SEM)
Age	64.7(1.5)
Education	13.7(1.1)
Verbal IQ[2]	110.5(8.2)
Performance IQ[2]	104.5(6.7)
Full Scale IQ[2]	108.2(7.9)
Impairment Index[4]	0.8(0.1)
WMSMQ[3]	92.3(10.1)

TABLE 2

	BASELINE MEAN(SEM)	PLACEBO MEAN(SEM)	FLUVOXAMINE MEAN(SEM)
DOPAC(pmol/ml)	2.8(0.5)	3.2(0.5)	3.6(0.6)
HVA(pmol/ml)	271.1(61.4)	211.1(41.4)	261.3(47.2)
5HIAA(pmol/ml)	128.1(25.5)	107.5(17.4)	71.5(12.4)
NE(pmol/ml)	0.5(0.1)	0.7(0.1)	0.8(0.3)
CRH(pg/ml)	57.5(13.0)	52.5(9.5)	47.0(6.8)
ACTH(pg/ml)	28.0(2.9)	26.1(1.5)	22.8(2.0)
DBI(pmol/ml) (Diazepam Binding Inhibitor)	1.6(0.2)	1.4(0.1)	1.4(0.1)
GNRH(pg/ml) (Gonadotropin-Releasing Hormone)	53.4(4.0)	56.3(3.4)	74.2(7.4)
NEUROPEPTIDE Y(pg/ml)	90.5(11.5)	101.5(11.3)	99.8(6.4)
SOMATOSTATIN(pg/ml)	83.7(14.8)	80.0(11.0)	71.8(13.3)
NEUROTENSIN(pg/200ul)	0.2(0.03)	0.2(0.03)	0.2(0.01)
MHPG-CSF(pmol/ml)	41.0(5.1)	36.9(3.6)	36.3(4.9)
MHPG-Plasma(pmol/ml)	15.5(1.5)	15.6(2.4)	14.9(2.2)

reuptake. No other changes between placebo and fluvoxamine conditions reached statistical significance with this small number of subjects.

Across the 6 patients, the change in CSF 5HIAA was not significantly correlated with the blood level of fluvoxamine ($r = -0.542$). The single dementia patient, however, was the only subject that failed to show noticeable change in CSF 5HIAA in spite of adequate blood levels of fluvoxamine. With this patient omitted, the relationship between blood level of fluvoxamine and change in CSF 5HIAA for the remaining 5 patients was statistically significant ($r = -0.906$, $p < .05$).

When all alcohol amnestic syndrome patients were considered as a group, fluvoxamine produced a small but significant improvement in episodic memory performance, resulting in an increase in free recall of words. Overall improvement in performance on the WMSMQ was associated with higher levels of fluvoxamine ($r = 0.80$, $p < .05$, one-tailed) and lower levels of 5HIAA ($r = -0.805$, $p < .05$, one-tailed). The two alcohol amnestic syndrome patients who had the highest blood levels of fluvoxamine demonstrated the largest changes in CSF 5HIAA and improvement in performance on WMSMQ under fluvoxamine.

DISCUSSION

These preliminary findings implicate a role of serotonergic mechanisms in alcoholic chronic organic brain syndrome. For alcoholic dementia, the data from a single patient suggest a lack of response to this serotonin reuptake inhibitor in terms of change in CSF 5HIAA. For alcohol amnestic syndrome, the patients can be readily sorted into two groups according to the measured blood levels of fluvoxamine. The two patients who showed blood levels of fluvoxamine of at least 200 ng/ml also showed large changes on CSF 5HIAA and an improvement in performance on WMSMQ under fluvoxamine. The three patients whose blood levels of fluvoxamine were less than 200 ng/ml showed negligible changes in CSF 5HIAA and WMSMQ. This finding suggests that with individual titration of the drug dose, fluvoxamine might be a clinically useful agent in the treatment of alcohol amnestic syndrome.

REFERENCES

1. Martin PR, Adinoff B, Weingartner H, Mukherjee AB, Eckardt MJ. Alcoholic organic brain disease: Nosology and pathophysiologic mechanisms. Prog Neuropsychopharmacol Biol Psychiatry. 1986; 10:147-164.

2. Matarazzo JD. Wechsler's measurement and appraisal of adult intelligence. Baltimore: Williams and Wilkins, 1972.

3. Prigatano GP. Wechsler Memory Scale: A selective review of the literature. J Clin Psychol. 1978; 34:816-832.

4. Boll TJ. The Halstead-Reitan Neuropsychological Battery. In: Filskov SB, Boll TJ, eds. Handbook of clinical neuropsychology. New York: Wiley, 1981:577-607.

5. Weingartner H, Rudorfer MU, Buchsbaum MS, Linnoila M. Effects of serotonin on memory impairments produced by ethanol. Science. 1983; 221:472-474.

Acute Effects of Ethanol on Motor Performance and Movement-Related Brain Potentials

John W. Rohrbaugh, PhD
June M. Stapleton, PhD
Henri W. Frowein, PhD
Bryon Adinoff, MD
Jerald L. Varner, PhD
Elizabeth A. Lane, PhD
Michael J. Eckardt, PhD
Markku Linnoila, MD, PhD

SUMMARY. The acute effects of ethanol on skilled motor functions were examined in male social drinkers, under four doses ranging from 0 (placebo) to 1.05 g/kg lean body weight. The movement entailed a forewarned choice transitive motion of the arm and hand, aimed at a flanking target. Performance measures disclosed only small effects of ethanol on speed and accuracy of movement. The simultaneously-recorded movement-related brain potentials disclosed decreased involvement of frontal and posterior brain areas, suggesting that ethanol disrupted the planning and regulation of movement despite the overall preservation of reaction speed.

It is often held that ethanol intoxication has negligible effects on reaction time (RT) and psychomotor performance, in contrast to its

---

The authors, with the exception of Henri W. Frowein, are affiliated with the Laboratory of Clinical Studies, Division of Intramural Clinical and Biological Research, National Institute on Alcohol Abuse and Alcoholism, NIH Clinical Center, Bldg. 10, Rm. 3C218, Bethesda, MD 20892. Henri W. Frowein is now with PTT Centrale Direktie, The Hague, The Netherlands.
Reprint requests should be sent to John W. Rohrbaugh.

pronounced effects on attention and cognition. A number of studies using the additive factor logic, however, have shown a consistent effect on RT, sometimes attributing the effect to a process of response selection. The present study examined the dose-related effects of ethanol in a situation entailing forewarned, aimed transitive movements of the hand and arm. Response measures were obtained separately for RT, and for movement time (MT). The RT and MT measures are held in the additive factors model to index response selection and response execution processes, respectively.[1] In addition, the accompanying brain electrical potentials were recorded during the warning period. These potentials consist of a complex of slow waves known collectively as the contingent negative variation (CNV). Although a number of variables combine to determine CNV amplitude, it is closely linked to movement parameters when a motor response is explicitly requested.[2]

The warned choice movement task entailed lifting a stylus from a central resting point and moving it to the left or right to contact a flanking target strip. The moment and direction of response were signalled by briefly illuminating one of two lateral lights. In one condition (S-R compatible) the correct response direction corresponded with stimulus location, whereas in a second condition (S-R incompatible) the direction was opposite. A warning signal, consisting of a compound light and tone stimulus, preceded the response signal by a warning period of 4 sec. Separate measures of RT (i.e., time to lift stylus from central point) and MT (i.e., subsequent time before contact with flanking strip) were obtained, as were measures of decision accuracy (i.e., direction of response) and movement precision (i.e., proportion of responses making contact with the target strip). Twelve subjects participated in a practice session plus four experimental sessions, each under a different dose and given in counterbalanced order. The ethanol doses were 0 (placebo), 0.45 (low), 0.80 (medium) and 1.05 (high) g/kg lean body weight, mixed in a constant volume with orange juice and consumed over a half-hour period. Additional maintenance doses of 0.12 g/kg were given at subsequent half-hour intervals. Data presented here were obtained in a run (which included both the compatible and incompatible conditions) starting 120 min after beginning of ethanol dosing, at which time the respective blood ethanol levels (as estimated by breath analysis) averaged 0, 37, 71 and 92 mg% for the four doses. The CNV was recorded with a long time constant from midline (Fpz, Fz, Cz, Pz and Oz) and lateral (C3, C4) placements, with reference to linked ear lobes.

Ethanol and S-R compatibility both affected RT, but there was no suggestion of an interaction between the two variables. RTs were lengthened 31 msec by S-R incompatibility, whereas at the highest dose ethanol increased RT by about 30 msec. The proportion of decision errors was low (averaging about 1%) and was not affected significantly as a function of dose or S-R compatibility. MT showed some reduction at the low dose and subsequent increase at higher doses, but these changes were over a total range of only 20 msec and were not statistically significant. Although about 20% of the movements were imprecise (i.e., did not make initial contact with the target strips), the rate was constant in the various conditions.

Grand averaged CNV waveforms under each dose, from the midline electrodes, are plotted in Figure 1. The early wave peaking at about 500 msec, which is related to the alerting properties of the warning signal,[2] was significantly enhanced under all ethanol doses. The late CNV wave was significantly affected by ethanol, although the effects were complex. At the central sites, ethanol produced a progressive but small reduction. More pronounced effects were obtained at the prefrontal and occipital sites (as indicated by a significant dose by site interaction), where the wave first increased slightly as a function of dose but showed a large decrement at the high dose. The positivity at Fpz under the high dose was a consistent effect, seen in all runs, for both compatible and incompatible responses, and for both left and right movements.

In sum, the effects of ethanol on performance measures were generally small. RT was significantly lengthened, by about 30 msec, but the lack of interaction between dose and S-R compatibility indicates that response selection processes were not affected. The small increase in MT indicates that response execution processes may be affected at higher doses, although the effect was extremely small and statistically non-significant. The effects of ethanol on the CNV were more appreciable, and were found to be opposite for early and late waves. This may explain why no net effect has sometimes been found with short warning periods,

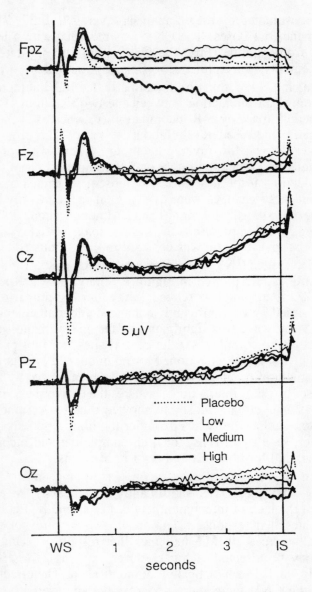

FIGURE 1. Brain electrical potentials recorded from midline electrodes during the interval between the warning stimulus (WS) and imperative stimulus (IS). Separate records are plotted for each dose.

wherein the waves may overlap. Prefrontal positivity preceding movement has previously been observed in very young and very old subjects.[3] The disproportionate reduction of the late CNV at prefrontal and posterior sites seen here with the high dose of ethanol may indicate a diminished participation of these areas, thought to be important for the planning and regulation of movement, despite the overall preservation of reaction speed.

REFERENCES

1. Frowein, H. W. Selective drug effects on human information processing. Soesterberg, The Netherlands: Institute for Perception TNO, 1981.

2. Rohrbaugh, J. W., and Gaillard, A. W. K. Sensory and motor aspects of the contingent negative variation. In: A. W. K. Gaillard and W. Ritter, eds., Tutorials in ERP Research: Endogenous Components. Amsterdam: North Holland, 1983: 269-310.

3. Deecke, L., Bashore, T., Brunia, C. H. M., Grunewald-Zuberbier, E., Grunewald, G. and Kristeva, R. Movement-associated potentials and motor control. In R. Karrer, J. Cohen and P. Tueting, eds., Brain and Information. Ann. N. Y. Acad. Sci., 1984; 425:398-428.

NEUROSCIENCE AND PSYCHOPHARMACOLOGY

Brain Imaging in Alcoholic Patients

Michael J. Eckardt, PhD
John W. Rohrbaugh, PhD
Daniel Rio, PhD
Robert R. Rawlings, MS
Richard Coppola, PhD

SUMMARY. Imaging *in vivo* aspects of brain structure and function hold great promise for the study of alcoholism. Computerized axial tomography and magnetic resonance imaging have been used successfully to demonstrate structural abnormalities in alcoholic patients. Positron emission tomography and topographic images of electrical and magnetic activity are useful measures of brain function that could be applied more rigorously to the study of alcoholism. Interrelating various types of imaging data is an important area that is still in the developmental stage.

Michael J. Eckardt, John W. Rohrbaugh, and Daniel Rio are affiliated with the Section of Clinical Brain Research, Laboratory of Clinical Studies, Division of Intramural Clinical and Biological Research, National Institute on Alcohol Abuse and Alcoholism, NIH Clinical Center, Bldg. 10, Rm. 3C218, Bethesda, MD 20892. Robert R. Rawlings is affiliated with the Division of Biometry and Epidemiology, NIAAA. Richard Coppola is affiliated with the National Institute of Mental Health.

Reprint requests should be directed to Michael J. Eckardt.

Recent developments in brain imaging techniques have fulfilled a long-existing need to visualize critical aspects of *in vivo* brain structure and function. The availability of imaging technology holds great promise for the study of alcoholism, as exemplified in recent symposia on the subject.[1,2] The intent of the present paper is to discuss selected imaging technologies and demonstrate how they are being used to investigate brain structure and function in alcoholics using chronic organic brain syndrome (OBS) as an example. This particular population of alcoholics is emphasized because severe OBS is a relatively common complication of alcoholism occurring in about 9% of alcoholics[3] and has been estimated to be the second most common cause of adult dementia (approximately 10%) following Alzheimer's disease (40-60%).[4] A description of our study has been published previously.[5]

STRUCTURE

Three different neuropathologic findings have been reported in chronic alcoholic patients: (1) cerebellar degeneration, (2) Wernicke's encephalopathy, and (3) reduction in brain weight.[6,7] Consequently, assessment of anatomy in the living brain is of importance for identifying pathological conditions as well as for conducting research on structure and function relationships. Anatomy of the living brain has been studied using radiologic (pneumoencephalography; computerized axial tomography—CAT; radionuclide cisternography) and magnetic (magnetic resonance imaging—MRI) methods.

Computerized Axial Tomography (CAT)

This radiologic method has been used widely in recent years to examine brain structure because of its relative ease, noninvasiveness, and high resolution (approximately 2 mm with present day instruments). Numerous CAT studies (with and without administration of contrast medium) of alcoholics have demonstrated sulcal enlargement, ventricular enlargement, and widened cerebellar folia.[8,9] Attempts to quantify CAT scans have met with variable success with fissural and sulcal enlargement being particularly difficult to measure accurately.[10] Various methods have been used to quantify ventricular size including linear measurements of the ventricular system, ratios of these measurements to internal cranial diameter (i.e., Evans ratio, frontal horn ratio, bicaudate ratio, cella media ratio), area of the ventricular system divided by the total area of the brain within a specific scan, and volumetric measurements computed from scans taken throughout the brain.[11] Although some investigators have derived estimates of tissue density from quantitative analysis of pixel values,[12-14] the value associated with each pixel can be influenced by measurement error associated with the instrument itself, patient motion, beam hardening, and partial volume effects. Moreover, additional sources of variability are introduced when studying more than one individual, including the selection of comparable scans, intra- and interobserver consistency, and alignment consistency.

Recent findings suggest that the widening of superficial sulci with age may be correlated with the loss of adjacent white matter,[15] and this coupled with the reported histological changes in white matter determined at autopsy in chronic alcoholics[16] emphasize the importance of differentiating among gray matter, white matter, and CSF in CAT scans. Although methods for solving this problem have been proposed, there is no clear agreement as yet.[17,18]

Several investigators have reported reversibility of CAT abnormalities in alcoholics with abstinence,[19-22] but the finding is not universal.[23] Moreover, the problems associated with realigning the patient in exactly the same position as on the first scan are complex and generally recognized as being a major impediment to accurate and reliable quantification.

One attempt to minimize the realignment problem is to construct three dimensional (3D) images. Appropriate reconstruction of 3D images enables the optimization of selecting CAT slices at similar levels across individuals. This approach also has the advantage of permitting volumetric analysis, thereby enabling more direct determination of the volume of specific structures within the cranial cavity. Of course, the importance of the mathematical assumptions inherent in constructing 3D images from a series of 2D images must not be minimized.

Magnetic Resonance Imaging (MRI)

MRI is a relatively new, noninvasive technique used to produce medical images. It is based on the principle that many naturally occurring nuclei have a magnetic moment and angular momentum associated with them. These nuclei are subjected to an applied static or stationary magnetic field characterized by a specific gradient. A subsequently applied radio frequency (RF) pulse of electromagnetic radiation will cause these nuclei to resonate. Since each nucleus occupies a different spatial position within the gradient magnetic field, each spatial volume will have a unique frequency associated with it, and the amplitude of the resonating signal will be proportional to the number of nuclei that are resonating. The most frequently chosen nuclei to excite are hydrogen because the resonant signal has a high signal-to-noise ratio (other nuclei which may be used are phosphorus and carbon). The technique that directly applies this methodology is called inversion-recovery, which makes use of a combination of applied gradients and a particular RF pulse sequence. Alternative pulsing arrangements, such as spin-echo technique, are possible which can extract additional or different information.

Information characterizing the environment in which the nuclei are situated is also carried by the resonating signal. This information is associated with the time required for the nuclei to relax back to their equilibrium state, denoted by T1, and to lose phase coherence, denoted by T2, after an application of a RF pulse. Techniques such as inversion-recovery or spin-echo may use this information to help differentiate white and gray matter in a brain image.

MRI has been found in many situations to be superior to CAT imaging, particularly for imaging subtentorial regions. Its resolution is equal to that of CAT (approximately 2 mm) and it involves no radiation. Moreover, MRI methodology has the enhanced capability of differentiating white and gray matter and fluid-filled ventricles. MRI has been used to describe global brain abnormalities in alcoholics,[24] and loss of structural integrity of the mamillary bodies in chronic Wernicke disease.[25] It has also been employed to measure brain water changes with abstinence in withdrawing alcoholics.[26]

FUNCTION

Functional integrity of the brain has been studied with a variety of approaches including neuropsychology,[27] positron emission tomography,[28] electroencephalography,[29] and magnetoencephalography.[30] Imaging techniques have been employed in the latter three.

Positron Emission Tomography (PET)

PET is a technique that offers a number of important research and clinical possibilities by allowing the precise quantification and localization in space of the extent to which positron-emitting radioactive isotopes are utilized in the brain. By measuring the local tissue concentrations of injected positron-emitting isotopes, 2D mathematical reconstructions of the rates of uptake in specific brain regions can be produced. Depending on the biological function of a particular isotope, different physiological processes can be investigated. The value of PET is that it allows for the study of physiological processes in the living brain. This technique thus complements neuroanatomical or histological measures of structure. PET also provides information on subcortical as well as cortical processes.

Oxygen[15] compounds have been used to study cerebral blood flow (CBF) and oxygen metabolism and fluorine[18]-deoxyglucose (FDG) has been used to study cerebral glucose utilization. Although CBF and glucose utilization may be related, the nature of this relationship may be disturbed in abnormal or pathophysiological conditions.[31]

Most PET studies have measured localized glucose metabolism using FDG as the radioactive tracer based on the models developed by Sokoloff et al.[32] and Reivich et al.[33] Since glucose is the primary energy source for the brain, resulting PET scan images quantify regional brain metabolism with the non-metabolized FDG. When the scanning (radiation detection) instrument is used to take a series of scans of successive planes of the brain, the images are topographically analogous to CAT or MRI scans, but reflect regional rates of glucose metabolism rather than anatomical detail.

Preliminary studies using PET have been conducted to investigate brain pathophysiology in alcoholic patients with chronic OBS. In the first study,[34] the mean cerebral glucose metabolic rate in long-term abstinent alcohol amnestic patients was found to be 22% lower than in age-matched normal controls when studied by PET (ECAT II scanner with average in-plane resolution of 17.5 mm) using FDG. Absolute rates of regional metabolism in these patients were significantly decreased in medial prefrontal and medial temporal cortical areas and in the thalamus and basal ganglia. Analysis of each subject's regional rates, relative to mean rate, revealed two distinct subgroups among the patients: those with (1) relatively low metabolism in anterior frontal cortex and relatively high activity in basal ganglia and thalamus, and (2) relatively high metabolism in the anterior frontal cortex and relatively low activity in the basal ganglia and thalamus. Dorsomedial parietal metabolism was relatively low in both subgroups. Clinically, both subgroups were amnestic, but the patients in the first subgroup appeared more demented. The identification of at least two patterns of cerebral metabolism in alcohol amnestic patients suggests different underlying neuropathologies, primarily cortical dysfunction in one and subcortical in the other.

In another PET study,[35] glucose metabolism in alcoholic OBS was compared with that in age-matched normal volunteers. Data were acquired with the NIH NeuroPet scanner (average in-plane resolution of 7 mm) in three sets of seven coplanar slices parallel to the canthomeatal plane. A preliminary region of interest (10 mm by 10 mm area) analysis of 18 symmetrical and 5 midline structures revealed no significant between-group differences in absolute rates of glucose metabolism, with the possible exception of the cerebellar vermis region. Multivariate discriminant analysis revealed conservative classification accuracies from 82 to 100%. Areas that best discriminated the groups were located in frontal cortex, cerebellar vermis, and third ventricle/hypothalamus. Although there are clear differences in results between these studies, one area of agreement is the involvement of the frontal cortex. This finding is supported further by a recent report of relatively decreased glucose metabolism in the medio-frontal cortex of a small sample of detoxified alcoholics without OBS.[36]

A rationale for obtaining 3D brain images of glucose utilization is similar to that developed for 3D analysis of CAT and MRI images including the advantages of direct volumetric analysis and improved realignment capabilities. Likewise, the mathematical assumptions of constructing 3D images from a series of 2D images need to be evaluated carefully.

Cerebral Blood Flow (CBF)

Although CBF studies can be conducted with PET methodology, resulting in similar imaging presentations, most of the studies involving alcoholics have been conducted with Xenon[133] which relies on a related, but somewhat different methodology.[37] In detoxified alcoholics, blood flow values have been reported generally to be decreased in gray matter[38] and in white matter as well in patients with Wernicke-Korsakoff syndrome.[38] Moreover, it is apparent that there are regional differences in magnitude of alcoholism-associated CBF alterations. Lastly, there have been reported improvements in CBF with abstinence and treatment.[37,38]

Electroencephalography (EEG) and Event-Related Brain Potentials (ERPs)

Electrical activity of the brain, when recorded at the scalp, represents the summed activity of large populations of cells. The principal sources are thought to be post-snypatic potentials generated in columnarly-organized cortical neurons, although activity from subcortical areas can be detected with some procedures. The composite signals are hybridized with contributions from glia and a variety of other non-neural sources. Unlike the other functional measures discussed above, an important aspect of electrical measures is the nature of changes over time, and indeed these electrical measures have typically provided some description of this temporal information in the form of signal frequency, wave shape, or latency. It has also long been recognized, however, that EEG and ERP signals also vary greatly as a function of where on the head the recordings are obtained, and that information about regional differences provides valuable clinical information with respect to localization of function. Although some of the localization uses of the EEG have been largely supplanted by alternative techniques described previously, recent developments underscore the tremendous amount of information, often untapped, available from systematic study of regional differences in electrical activity.

Several technical considerations apply to the study of spatial aspects of brain electrical activity. Given the practical limitations of electrode size and number of amplification channels available, the electrical signals are typically recorded from an array of sites separated from one another by several centimeters. Although the resultant spatial resolution compares unfavorably with other techniques described previously, it is compatible with the nature of the electrical signals which are generated some distance from the scalp and distributed widely when conducted by volume through the intervening tissue.

A convenient method for displaying the spatial character of a given signal is to construct a topographic map in which some pertinent value is plotted as a function of spatial position. Such maps can be generated to depict activity within various frequency bands, or to describe other features of the signal such as instantaneous amplitude.[39] Various aspects of brain electrical activity have been related to such factors as selection of measurement sites, inter-electrode distances, spatial interpolation algorithms, control for artifact, and display factors and are discussed elsewhere.[40]

The systematic study of topographic information offers a number of advantages. One advantage is that topographic information is often taken to provide a defining characteristic of certain EEG patterns or ERP components. Topographic information may also serve as the basis for description of dynamic patterns of interrelationships among brain regions.[41,42] Perhaps most importantly, topographic distributional data may provide information with respect to the underlying brain sources and the extent to which they are affected by various clinical or experimental factors.

There are a number of findings which indicate that the spatial distribution of EEG and ERP signals is affected by alcohol.[43] Although these effects have not been systematically studied using

EEG/ERP imaging techniques, the previously mentioned considerations would suggest that this may be a profitable matter for study.

Magnetoencephalography (MEG)

Additional information regarding electrophysiological activity in various regions of the brain can be obtained from study of the magnetic counterpart of the electrical response. Such activity can be measured using a SQUID (superconducting quantum interference device) to detect the extremely small magnetic fields associated with current flow in brain tissue. When such activity is measured from multiple sites about the head, a map depicting the field distribution can be constructed in a manner similar to that described previously for electrical measurements.[30] The maps associated with both types of recording technique are systematically related to the nature of the electromotive source. The magnetic data, however, offer several unique features. One is that the MEG technique is particularly good for determining the location of unknown sources. This is because the meninges, skull, and scalp tissue do not greatly affect the distribution of the magnetic fields detected superficially, so that source depth, location, and orientation can be determined. Another advantage is that the magnetic technique yields data that are complementary and nonredundant with those recorded electrically. Whereas the electrical response seen at the scalp derives primarily from extracellular current flow in sources oriented radially to the scalp, the magnetic response appears to derive from intracellular current flow in tangentially-oriented sources. Despite these theoretical advantages, however, there are a number of practical limitations, particularly when distributed or multiple sources contribute to the field.[44] Although the MEG technique would appear to offer considerable promise for the study of alcoholism, we are not aware of any such studies conducted to date.

INTERRELATIONSHIPS AMONG IMAGING DATA

Structure-function relationships and comparison among different types of functional measures are intrinsically interesting but difficult because of differing instruments and associated technologies. Our own studies are designed to use a variety of complementary techniques described previously for evaluating brain function and structure.[5] This is to be accomplished by evaluating the pathophysiology identified by PET, referring it to the brain morphology measured by CAT and MRI, and supplementing these data with measures of brain electrical activity and cognition. Each of these individually selected measures has been shown previously to provide useful information on alcoholism-related brain dysfunction: PET,[35] CAT,[9] MRI,[24] EEG,[29] and neuropsychology.[27]

REFERENCES

1. Chao HM, Foudin L. Symposium on imaging research in alcoholism. Alcohol Clin Exp Res. 1986; 10:223-225.

2. Chao HM. NIAAA/ARUS Symposium entitled "Imaging Research in Alcoholism II." San Francisco, 1986.

3. Horvath TB. Clinical spectrum and epidemiological features of alcoholic dementia. In: Rankin JG, ed. Alcohol, drugs and brain damage. Toronto: Addiction Research Foundation, 1975: 1-16.

4. Wells CE. Diagnosis of dementia. Psychosomatics 1979; 20:517-522.

5. Johnson JL, Adinoff B, Bisserbe JC, Martin PR, Rio D, Rohrbaugh JW, Zubovic E, Eckardt MJ. Assessment of alcoholism-related organic brain syndromes with positron emission tomography. Alcohol Clin Exp Res. 1986; 10:237-240.

6. Victor M, Laureno R. Neurologic complications of alcohol abuse: epidemiologic aspects. In: Schoenberg BS, ed. Advances in neurology. New York: Raven Press, 1978: 603-616.

7. Torvik A, Lindboe CF, Roade S. Brain lesions in alcoholics: a neuropathological study with clinical correlations. J Neurol Sci. 1982; 56:233-248.

8. Cala LA, Mastaglia FL. Computerized tomography in chronic alcoholics. Alcohol Clin Exp Res. 1981; 5:283-294.

9. Wilkinson DA. Examination of alcoholics by computed tomographic (CT) scans: a critical review. Alcohol Clin Exp Res. 1982; 6:31-45.

10. Turkheimer E, Cullum CM, Hubler DN, Paver SN, Yeo RA, Bigler ED. Quantifying cortical atrophy. J Neurol Neurosurg Psychiatry 1984; 47:1314-1318.

11. LeMay M. Radiologic changes of the aging brain and skull. AJR 1984; 143:383-389.

12. Carlen PL, Wilkinson DA. Alcoholic brain damage and reversible deficits. Acta Psychiatr Scand. 1980; 62 (Suppl 286):103-118.

13. Golden CJ, Grabler B, Blose I, Berg R, Coffman J, Block S. Difference

in brain densities between chronic alcoholics and normal control patients. Science 1981; 211:508-510.

14. Gebhardt CA, Naeser MA, Butters N. Computerized measures of CT scans of alcoholics: thalamic region related to memory. Alcohol 1984; 1:133-140.

15. Miller AKH, Alston RL, Corsellis JAN. Variations with age in the volume of grey and white matter in the cerebral hemispheres of man: measurements with an image analyser. Neuropathol Appl Neurobiol. 1980; 6:119-132.

16. Harper CG, Krill JJ, Holloway RL. Brain shrinkage in chronic alcoholics: a pathological study. Brit Med J. 1985; 290:501-505.

17. DeLee JM, Schwartz M, Creasey H, Cutler N, Rapoport SI. Computer-assisted categorization of brain computerized tomography pixels into cerebrospinal fluid, white matter, and gray matter. Comput Biomed Res. 1985; 18:79-88.

18. Pfefferbaum A, Zatz LM, Jernigan TL. Improved computer-interactive method for quantifying cerebrospinal fluid and tissue in brain CT scans: effects of aging. J Comput Assist Tomogr. 1986; 10:571-578.

19. Carlen PL, Wilkinson DA, Wortzman G, Holgate RC. Partially reversible cerebral atrophy and functional improvement in abstinent alcoholics. Can J Neuroradiol. 1984; 11:441-446.

20. Artmann H, Gall MV, Hacker H, Herrlick J. Reversible enlargement of cerebral spinal fluid spaces in chronic alcoholics. Am J Neuroradiol. 1981; 2:23-27.

21. Ron MA, Acker W, Shaw GK, Lishman WA. Computerized tomography of the brain in chronic alcoholics: a survey and follow-up study. Brain 1982; 105:497-514.

22. Cala LA, Jones B, Burns P, Davis RE, Stenhouse N, Mastaglia FL. Results of computerized tomography, psychometric testing and dietary studies in social drinkers, with emphasis on reversibility after abstinence. Med J Aust. 1983; 2:264-269.

23. Hill SY, Mikhael M. Computed tomography scans of alcoholics: cerebral atrophy? Science 1979; 204:1237-1238.

24. Besson JAO, Glen AIM, Foreman EI, MacDonald A, Smith FW, Hutchinson JMS, Mallard JR, Ashcroft GW. Nuclear magnetic resonance observations in alcoholic cerebral disorder and the role of vasopressin. Lancet 1981; 2:923-924.

25. Charness ME, DeLaPaz RL. Mamillary body atrophy in Wernicke's encephalopathy. Antemortem identification using magnetic resonance imaging. Ann Neurol. 1987; 22:595-600.

26. Smith MA, Chick J, Kean DM, Douglas RHB, Singer A, Kendall RE, Bert JJK. Brain water in chronic alcoholic patients measured by magnetic resonance imaging. Lancet 1985; 1:1273-1274.

27. Eckardt MJ, Martin PR. Clinical assessment of cognition in alcoholism. Alcohol Clin Exp Res. 1986; 10:123-127.

28. Phelps M, Mazziotta J, Huang S. Study of cerebral function with positron computed tomography. J Cereb Blood Flow Metab. 1982; 2:113-167.

29. Spehr N, Stemmler G. Postalcoholic diseases: diagnostic relevance of computerized EEG. Electroenceph clin Neurophysiol. 1985; 60:106-114.

30. Weinberg H, Brickett P, Robertson A, Harrop R, Cheyne DO, Crisp D, Baff M, Dykstra C. The magnetoencephalographic localization of source-systems in the brain: early and late components of event related potentials. In: Rohrbaugh JW, Begleiter H, eds. Alcohol and event-related brain potentials. Alcohol 1987; 4:339-345.

31. Fox PT, Raichle ME. Focal physiological uncoupling of cerebral blood flow and oxidative metabolism during somatosensory stimulation in human subjects. Proc Natl Acad Sci. 1986; 83:1140-1144.

32. Sokoloff L, Reivich M, Kennedy C, DesRosiers MH, Patlak CS, Pettigrew KD, Sakuraja O, Shinohara M. The [^{14}C] deoxyglucose method for the measurement of local cerebral glucose utilization: theory, procedure, and normal values in the conscious and anesthetized albino rat. J Neurochem. 1977; 28:897-916.

33. Reivich M, Alair A, Greenberg J, Fowler J, Christman D, Wolf A, Rosenquist A, Hand P. Metabolic mapping of functional cerebral activity in man using ^{18}F-2-fluoro-2-deoxyglucose technique. J Comput Assist Tomogr. 1979; 2:656-665.

34. Kessler RM, Parker ES, Clark CM, Martin PR, George DT, Weingartner H, Sokoloff L, Ebert MN, Mishkin M. Regional cerebral glucose metabolism in patients with alcoholic Korsakoff's syndrome. Soc Neuroscience Abstr. 1984; 10:541.

35. Martin PR. PET studies of alcoholic chronic organic brain syndrome. Presented at NIAAA/ARUS sponsored symposium entitled "Imaging Research in Alcoholism II." San Francisco, CA, 1986.

36. Samson Y, Baron JC, Feline A, Borles J, Crouzel C. Local cerebral glucose utilisation in chronic alcoholics: a positron tomographic study. J Neurol Neurosurg Psychiat. 1986; 49:1165-1170.

37. Meyer JS, Tanahashi N, Ishikawa Y, Hata T, Velez M, Fann WE, Kandula P, Mortel KF, Rogers RL. Cerebral atrophy and hypoperfusion improvement during treatment of Wernicke-Korsakoff syndrome. J Cereb Blood Flow Metabol. 1985; 5:376-385.

38. Ishikawa Y, Meyer JS, Tanahasi N, Hata T, Velez M, Fann WE, Kandula P, Motel KF, Rogers RL. Abstinence improves cerebral perfusion and brain volume in alcoholic neurotoxicity without Wernicke-Korsohoff syndrome. J Cereb Blood Flow Metabol. 1986; 6:86-94.

39. Coppola, R. Isolating low frequency components in EEG spectrum analysis. Electroenceph clin Neurophysiol. 1978; 46:224-226.

40. Coppola R. Issues in topographic analysis of EEG activity. In: Duffy FH, ed. Topographic mapping of brain electrical activity. Boston: Butterworths, 1986: 339-346.

41. Duffy FH. Brain electrical activity mapping: issues and answers. In: Duffy FH, ed. Topographic mapping of brain electrical activity. Boston: Butterworths, 1986: 401-419.

42. Gevins A. Analysis of multiple lead data. In: Rohrbaugh JW, Johnson R, Parasuraman R, eds. Interdisciplinary vantages in event-related potential research. New York: Oxford, in press.

43. Rohrbaugh JW and Begleiter H. eds. Alcohol and Event-Related Potentials. Alcohol 1987; 4:223-224.

44. Nunez PL. The brain's magnetic field: some effects of multiple sources on localization methods. Electroenceph clin Neurophysiol. 1986; 63:75-82.

Pharmacology of Alcohol Preference in Rodents

Ting-Kai Li, MD
Lawrence Lumeng, MD
William J. McBride, PhD
James M. Murphy, PhD
Janice C. Froehlich, PhD
Sandra Morzorati, PhD

SUMMARY. In alcoholism research, two fundamental and closely related questions are: "Why do people drink?" and "Why do some people drink too much?" Humans voluntarily drink alcoholic beverages or self-administer alcohol, more often than not, in a social setting. Environmental factors and how individuals react to them can, therefore, have powerful influences on drinking behavior. On the other hand, the neuropsychopharmacological actions of ethanol and how different individuals react to them can be important biological determinants. Ethanol's action is biphasic, i.e., it can be reinforcing (rewarding) in the low concentration range, but aversive at high concentrations.[1] Perception by the individual of the reinforcing actions of ethanol might be expected to maintain alcohol-seeking behavior, whereas aversive effects would be expected to extinguish this behavior. Identification of the environmental and biological variables that promote and maintain alcohol-seeking or alcohol self-administration behavior is key to our understanding of the disorder alcoholism itself.

The authors are affiliated with The Regenstrief and Psychiatric Research Institutes, Departments of Medicine, Psychiatry and Biochemistry, Indiana University School of Medicine, 1110 West Michigan Street, Indianapolis, IN 46202, and the Veterans Administration Medical Center.

Reprint requests should be sent to Ting-Kai Li.

This research was supported in part by PHS AA-03243.

73

There is now a large body of literature describing possible psychosocial antecedents or risk factors of problem drinking. Sociocultural norms, family environment, peer-group influences and stages of psychosocial development are among some of the factors that can promote the initiation of drinking, as well as its continuation and progression. Changes in life events and development of problems can encourage moderation or cessation. By contrast, relatively little is known about specific biological processes and pathways that promote problem drinking and alcoholism in humans. However, there is now convincing evidence for identifiable genetic risk in a large segment of the alcoholic population.[2,3] Thus, there is biological predisposition for "drinking too much" in some individuals, and what this inherited propensity (or propensities) might be is currently a subject of intense clinical research interest.

In looking at various biological responses to ethanol that can serve as feedback loops to influence alcohol drinking behavior in humans, it is noteworthy that a number of them, as well as drinking behavior itself, have shown a large degree of between-individual variability that is, in part, genetically determined.[4,5] These include: alcohol elimination rate, the sensitivity of the brain to the action of alcohol, as exemplified by patterns of ethanol-induced change in the electroencephalogram, and systemic reactivity to ethanol metabolism, as evidenced by the alcohol-flush reaction. Although specific studies have yet to be performed, it can be expected that several other kinds of responses of the brain to alcohol's actions would be influenced by genetic factors. These include: (a) individual differences in sensitivity to the reinforcing effects of ethanol (b) individual differences in capacity for developing tolerance to the aversive effects of ethanol, and (c) individual differences in severity of withdrawal reactions owing to physical dependence.

Experiments on the heritability of the high dose aversive effects of ethanol and of the chronic effects of ethanol administration (tolerance and physical dependence) are difficult to justify in humans for ethical reasons. Such studies and the study of the relation of these responses to alcohol-seeking behavior are more appropriately carried out in laboratory animals. In this context, if alcoholism is defined as a disorder of abnormally intense alcohol-seeking behavior that over time leads to the alcohol dependence syndrome,[6] it becomes amenable to experimental study. Since alcohol-seeking behavior is the final common pathway in alcoholism, regardless of etiology, exploration of its neuroanatomical, neurophysiological and neurochemical substrates is key to our understanding of the biology of this disorder.

A GENETIC APPROACH TO DEVELOPING ANIMAL MODELS FOR ALCOHOLISM RESEARCH

Over the years, a number of investigators have attempted to develop suitable animal models for laboratory study. In a recent review,[7] the kinds of criteria that an animal model of alcoholism should ideally satisfy were discussed, and the limitations of the animal models then extant were evaluated. With the realization that the sociocultural and psychosocial variables that influence drinking behavior in humans cannot be incorporated into an animal model, the following criteria have been proposed:

1. The animal must self-administer ethanol in pharmacologically significant amounts. Specifically, the following conditions must be met:

   a. ethanol should be self-administered by oral intake,
   b. ethanol should be consumed preferentially when there is a choice between it and another equally palatable fluid or water,
   c. consumption should give rise to pharmacologically meaningful blood alcohol concentrations (BACs),
   d. voluntary intake should be based on its pharmacological effects, not because of its caloric value, taste, or smell.

2. Tolerance to ethanol should be demonstrable following a period of continuous consumption. Specifically, animals should be less affected in performance by the same dose and blood level of ethanol after a period of chronic exposure.

3. Dependence on ethanol should develop after a period of continuous consumption. Physical dependence is measured by characteristic behavioral and physiological signs during acute

ethanol withdrawal. Although psychological or behavioral dependence in the human sense of the term cannot be elicited from an animal, its operant behavior to ethanol as a "reinforcer" can provide a measure of abuse liability or reinforcing efficacy of the substance for that animal. When ethanol is able to maintain operant responding, behavioral dependence is assumed to have occurred.

Most species of laboratory animals do not exhibit a liking for unadulterated aqueous solutions containing moderate to high concentrations of ethanol. An obvious reason is that most animals do not like the taste of moderately concentrated alcoholic solutions, despite its potentially reinforcing properties. Parenthetically, most humans do not particularly enjoy the taste of unchilled alcoholic solutions either, since they have gone to great lengths to disguise the taste of alcohol in alcoholic beverages.

A number of approaches to increasing oral consumption of ethanol in experimental animals have been explored;[8] the most successful of these has been genetic. McClearn and Rodgers[9] first showed that inbred strains of mice differed widely in their preference for a 10% solution of ethanol versus water. Differences among inbred strains in a trait may be regarded as prima facie evidence of a genetic influence on that trait. Capitalizing on this genetic potential, a number of rat lines that differ in alcohol preference have been developed through selective breeding. Selective breeding is the process by which individuals who exhibit the most extreme levels of a chosen phenotype (e.g., high and low voluntary alcohol consumption) are mated in successive generations. Over time, the selected lines would have a high or low frequency of the genes that impact on that trait, while the frequency of the genes not affecting that trait should remain randomly distributed. These pharmacogenetically different animal lines provide useful tools for investigating mechanisms, since associated traits are likely to share common mechanisms through common gene action.

There currently are three pairs (high and low) of established rat lines that differ in alcohol preference, developed through selective breeding from different foundation stocks. The first of these, the UChA (low preference) and the UChB (high preference) lines were developed in Chile.[10] Subsequently, the high preference AA and low preference ANA lines were established in Finland.[11] The third set, the high preference P and the low preference NP lines were developed in our laboratory.[12]

The P and NP lines were developed through mass selection for high and low alcohol preference from a foundation stock of Wistar rats.[13] Testing was performed with an unflavored 10% (v/v) solution of ethanol made continuously available in a Richter tube to individually housed animals. Water in an identical Richter tube as an alternate source of fluid and solid food were provided *ad libitum*. The amounts of 10% ethanol, water and food consumed daily were measured for three weeks, and those animals exhibiting the highest and lowest consumption scores (g ethanol/kg body weight/d) were mated to initiate subsequent generations of P and NP lines, respectively. After 20 generations, the consumption scores (g/kg/d; mean ± SD) were: P males, 5.5 ± 1.2; P females, 7.3 ± 1.7; NP males, 1.1 ± 0.6; NP females 1.0 ± 0.9. The consumption scores in the current S26 and S27 generations are: P males, 6.2 ± 1.5; P females 7.0 ± 2.1; NP males, 0.9 ± 0.7; and NP females, 1.4 ± 0.2. More recently, we have begun a second selection experiment for high and low alcohol drinking preference from a more heterogeneous foundation stock, the N/Nih,[14] with use of within family selection and a rotational breeding design to minimize inbreeding. The duplicate high (HAD) and low (LAD) lines are now in the 6th generation of selection, and their drinking scores (g/kg/d) are HAD-1, 4.6 ± 2.3; LAD-1, 1.3 ± 1.1; HAD-2, 3.9 ± 2.0; LAD-2, 1.07 ± 0.28.

The P line of rats has now been systematically characterized with respect to the criteria described above for an animal model of alcoholism. With food, water and a 10% solution of ethanol available *ad libitum*, the P rats consume between 20-30% of the total calories as ethanol, and substitute ethanol calories for a part of the food calories. Weight gain is the same as in the control animals not given the ethanol solution as a fluid choice.[15] The P rats consume about 70% of the ethanol in the dark, when they also eat most of the food. Drinking occurs in bursts at irregularly-spaced intervals,[16] and some animals take in as much as 2-3 g ethanol/kg body weight in a single drinking episode. When blood is sampled five minutes after the completion of observed drinking episodes, BACs ranging between 43-122 mg% have been obtained; mean values are about 65 mg%.[12,17] At one hour after observed drinking episodes, BACs are 42-218 mg%; mean is 87 mg%.[18] Clearly, these animals are attaining systemic alcohol concentrations that are pharmacologically active, at least for humans. Notably, BACs of 50-70 mg% produced by intravenous infusion leads to curtailment of oral intake.[19] Therefore, the reinforcing action of ethanol for the P rats appears to occur at concentrations below 100 mg%, and the higher BACs attained after drinking have ceased represent overshoot, caused by delayed gastrointestinal absorption.

With chronic free-choice drinking of 10% ethanol, the P rats develop behavioral or neuronal tolerance as assessed by a jump-out test.[20] It was found that after 14 days of free-choice drinking, the P rats exhibited neuronal tolerance, since they required a shorter time to recover to criterion performance and BACs were higher at time of recovery.[21] In separate experiments, the P rats also were shown to develop metabolic tolerance with chronic free-choice drinking of 10% ethanol. After six weeks, ethanol elimination rate of the ethanol-consuming animals was 15% higher than that of the control animals.[17] Weight gain and total caloric intake of the animals were identical in the two groups. It has also been demonstrated that chronic free-choice drinking by the P rats produces physical dependence.[16] Experimental animals were given constant access to 10% ethanol and water for 20 weeks, while control animals received only water. Food was available *ad libitum*. After 20 weeks, the ethanol solution was taken away from the experimental animals and, in the first 24 hours following the removal of ethanol, 18 of the 19 ethanol-exposed animals exhibited signs of withdrawal which abated within 72 hours. As expected, none of the control animals showed withdrawal signs.

We showed early on in our studies that the P rats will work to obtain ethanol through operant responding.[22] In fact, response rates of over 1,000 bar-presses/24 hours were obtained in each of the animals tested. Since food and water were freely available to the animals, it seemed unlikely that the P animals found the ethanol solutions rewarding because of caloric needs or thirst. In sharp contrast, rats unselected for ethanol preference would not bar-press for ethanol as reward unless they had been weight-reduced and restricted in caloric intake.[23] The oral ethanol self-administration behavior of the P rats also has been examined in a two-lever operant design, with water and different concentrations of ethanol in water as the alternate reinforcers. Food was made available *ad libitum*. The P rats self-administered more of the ethanol solution than water even when ethanol concentration was raised to 30%. With 15% and 20% ethanol, they self-administered between 8.5 and 9.5 g ethanol/kg per day. These amounts are higher than what they normally drink out of Richter tubes at these ethanol concentrations, suggesting that work increases the salience of ethanol as a reinforcer for the P rats. By contrast, NP rats showed a preference for water was soon as the ethanol solution exceeded 5%.

The above studies could not distinguish whether the reinforcing properties of ethanol for the P rats arise from its systemic actions or from its taste and smell. To demonstrate that the post-ingestive effects of ethanol are reinforcing to the P rats, intragastric ethanol self-administration experiments were performed, using the experimental design reported by Deutsch and co-workers.[24,25] It was found that, with food freely available throughout the experiment, the P rats consistently self-infused greater volumes of 10, 20, 30 and 40% (v/v) solutions of ethanol and lesser volumes of water than did the NP rats.[26] The amounts of ethanol infused by the NP rats were less than 1 g/kg/d at all concentrations of ethanol tested, whereas the amount of ethanol infused by the P rats increased from 3.0 ± 0.3 g/kg/d with 10% ethanol to 9.4 ± 1.7 g/kg/d with 40% ethanol. The BACs of animals measured 30 minutes after observed episodes of ethanol self-infusion of 20% ethanol were 100-400 mg%. All animals repeatedly showed signs of intoxication. The BACs attained with intragastric self-administration were considerably higher than those observed in the P rats with free-choice drinking, suggesting that orosensory cues may be an important modulator of ethanol drinking.

It is important to note that Deutsch and Eisner[27] were able to demonstrate intragastric self-administration of large amounts of ethanol in rats unselected for ethanol preference only if the rats had first been made physically dependent by the prior, forcible administration of ethanol. Ethanol self-administration behavior was quickly extinguished in unselected animals not made ethanol-dependent, as was observed in this study also with the NP rats. By contrast, the P animals in this study had not been made dependent on ethanol and, in fact, were ethanol-free for at least a month before the experiments. Clearly, the innate ethanol preference of experimental animals is an important — if not crucial — variable in studies of ethanol self-administration, as well as in efforts to establish an oral consumption animal model of alcoholism.

DIFFERENCES IN RESPONSE TO LOW AND HIGH DOSE ETHANOL BETWEEN THE P AND NP RATS

The findings summarized previously indicate that the P line of selectively-bred rats should be a useful animal model for elucidating the biology of alcohol-seeking behavior and for exploring conditions and agents that lessen this kind of behavior. Furthermore, they suggest that ethanol at concentrations below 100 mg% is reinforcing to the P rats and that ethanol at high concentrations may be more aversive to the NP rats than to the P rats. A number of studies have been performed to examine these relationships.

The P rats are innately more active than the NP rats,[12] and they exhibit increased spontaneous motor activity (SMA) following the intraperitoneal injection of ethanol, 0.1 to 0.5 g/kg body weight. BACs achieved with these doses are about 15-75 mg%. By contrast, the NP rats do not manifest stimulation at all. The increase in SMA in the P rats is as much as 50% with repeated daily injections of ethanol, 0.25 g/kg. No tolerance or reverse tolerance was observed over seven days.[28] In support of a difference between P and NP rats in response to low-dose ethanol, a differential effect on EEG activity during non-REM sleep has been observed in the P and NP rats after intragastric administration of ethanol, 0.5 g/kg body weight. With EEG electrodes implanted in the frontal cortex and dorsal hippocampus, the P rats showed a consistent decrease in power across all frequency bands, whereas power in the NP rats was consistently increased. This differential effect was evident 0-10 minutes and 30-40 minutes after ethanol administration at which time the BACs average 32 ± 4 mg% and 18 ± 4 mg%, respectively.[29]

Striking differences in response to higher doses of ethanol have also been observed between the P and NP lines. The NP rats manifest suppression of spontaneous locomotor activity at a lower dose of ethanol (1.0 g/kg) than do the P rats, and the P rats develop acute (within-session) tolerance to the high-dose, sedative-hypnotic effects of ethanol more quickly than do NP rats.[30] Even more interestingly, acute tolerance developed in the P rats to a single dose of ethanol can persist for as long as 10 days, whereas tolerance dissipated within three days in the NP rats.[31] A similar difference has been observed between the HAD and LAD rats.[32] It is of interest that the most robust association of high voluntary alcohol consumption thus far discovered in animal studies has been acute tolerance development. In addition to the P and NP rats and the HAD and LAD rats, this association has been seen in comparing the alcohol-preferring C57BL and the alcohol-nonpreferring DBA mouse strains,[33] in the HS/Ibg (heterogeneous stock) mice,[34] and in the selectively-bred, alcohol-preferring AA and the alcohol-nonpreferring ANA rats.[35]

The dose-dependent, reinforcing and aversive actions of ethanol were recently examined in the P and NP rats in a conditioned taste aversion study.[36] Injections of different concentrations of ethanol were paired with the drinking of saccharin solution, and the animals were then tested for drinking preference in a choice between the saccharin solution and water. Interestingly, with a low dose of ethanol (0.25 g/kg) the P rats exhibited conditioned facilitation, whereas the NP rats showed no effect. At the 1.0 g/kg dose, NP rats began to show conditioned aversion to drinking the saccharin solution, but the P rats were unaffected. With larger doses, e.g., 2.0 g/kg, ethanol produced conditioned aversion in both the P and NP rats. These experiments are consistent with the notion that: (a) low-dose ethanol is rewarding to the P rats, but not to the NP rats, and (b) the P rats are less affected than are the NP rats by the high-dose aversive actions of ethanol.

The combination of an enhanced response to the low-dose stimulatory and/or rewarding effects of ethanol and the rapid development of acute tolerance to the high-dose aversive effects of ethanol which persists over a long period of time provides an attractive hypothesis for explaining propensity towards alcohol abuse. As tolerance to the high-dose effects of ethanol develops, the rewarding actions of ethanol become progressively extended into the high blood alcohol concentration range, leading to increased consumption. We currently are testing this hypothesis in the P line of rats and are looking at neurohumoral concomitants of these effects.

NEUROCHEMICAL AND NEUROPHARMACOLOGICAL DIFFERENCES BETWEEN ETHANOL-NAIVE P AND NP RATS

A major discovered neurochemical difference between the P and NP lines is in the regional brain content of serotonin (5-HT). Ethanol-naive P rats have consistently exhibited lower levels of serotonin in the cerebral cortex, corpus striatum, thalamus, hypothalamus and hippocampus, and lower levels of 5-hydroxyindole acetic acid (5-HIAAA) in the cerebral cortex and hippocampus, than do ethanol-naive NP rats.[37] Less consistently, a lower content of norepinephrine (NE) and dopamine (DA) has been found in certain brain regions of P than of NP rats, e.g., NE in cortex and pons-medulla and DA in cortex. Differences in GABA and other putative amino acid neurotransmitters, e.g., Glu, Asp, Ala and Gly, have not been observed between the ethanol-naive P and NP animals. We also have measured the regional brain monoamine contents of alcohol-preferring and alcohol-nonpreferring animals in the N/Nih heterogeneous stock rats. The principal finding was a lowered content of DA and NE in the thalamus of the alcohol-preferring animals.[38] These observations strengthen the relevance of the association between brain 5-HT and alcohol drinking behavior.

In a recent study, we found that the nucleus accumbens of the P rats has lower levels of 5-HT, 5-HIAA, DA, dihydroxyphenylacetic acid and homovanillic acid.[39] The frontal cortex of the P rats also has decreased 5-HT and 5-HIAA. Since the nucleus accumbens and frontal cortex are important structures in brain reward circuitry, the decreased 5-HT, DA and metabolites suggest that the P rats have a specific deficiency of serotonergic projections from the dorsal raphe nucleus and of dopaminergic projections from the ventral tegmental area to these brain structures. In another study, we have observed that the binding of ^{3}H-5-HT to 5-HT$_1$ receptors in membranes of cerebral cortex and hippocampus is significantly higher in density (Bmax) and affinity (lower Kd) in the P than in the NP rats.[40] Since these brain regions of the P rats are low in 5-HT, the higher Bmax values and lower Kd values most likely reflect up-regulation and supersensitivity of 5HT$_1$ receptors as a compensatory mechanism to the lowered presynaptic input of 5-HT. Further support for the involvement of the serotonin neuronal pathways in ethanol preference has come from neuropharmacological studies. Fluoxetine and fluvoxamine, both relatively specific serotonin reuptake inhibitors, have been found to be effective in reducing voluntary ethanol consumption in the P rats both on a 24-hour, free-choice, oral consumption schedule and with intragastric ethanol self-administration.[41,42] The lowering of alcohol intake occurs with doses of drug that do not significantly affect water and food in the P rats.

While the evidence implicates an association between high alcohol preference and decreased density and/or metabolic functioning of the 5-HT neuronal system, it is unlikely that an abnormality in a single transmitter system determines alcohol preference. Indeed, desipramine (a NE reuptake inhibitor) also curtails alcohol preference in the P rats, and naloxone inhibits alcohol drinking the HAD line of rats.[43] Preliminary data suggest that HAD rats have higher levels of met-enkephalin in the hypothalamus and in the anterior and posterior striatum than LAD rats.[43] Ongoing studies are aimed at elucidating the nature of the interactions of these neurotransmitter systems in alcohol preference.

REFERENCES

1. Pohorecky LA. Biphasic action of ethanol. Biobehav Rev. 1977; 1:231-240.

2. Cloninger CR, Bohman M, Sigvardsson S. Inheritance of alcohol abuse: cross-fostering analysis of adopted men. Arch Gen Psychiatry. 1981; 38:861-868.

3. Bohman M, Sigvardsson S, Cloninger CR. Maternal inheritance of alcohol abuse: cross-fostering analysis of adopted women. Arch Gen Psychiatry. 1981; 38:965-969.

4. Li T-K. Genetic variability in response to ethanol in humans and experimental animals. In: Towle LH, ed. NIAAA-WHO Collaborating Center Designa-

tion Meeting and Alcohol Research Seminar. Washington, DC: U.S. Government Printing Office, 1985:50-62.

5. McClearn GE, Erwin VG. Mechanisms of genetic influence on alcohol-related behaviors. In: Alcohol and Health Monograph I. Alcohol Consumption and Related Problems. Washington, DC: U.S. Government Printing Office, 1982:263-289.

6. Edwards G, Gross, MM. Alcohol dependence: provisional description of a clinical syndrome. Br Med J. 1976; 1:1058-1061.

7. Cicero TJ. A critique of animal analogues of alcoholism. In: Majchrowicz, Noble EP, eds. Biochemistry and Pharmacology of Ethanol. New York: Plenum Press, 1979; 2:533-560.

8. Deitrich RA, Melchior CL. A critical assessment of animal models for testing new drugs for altering ethanol intake. In: Naranjo CA, Sellers EM, eds. Research Advances in New Psychopharmacological Treatments for Alcoholism. Amsterdam, Netherlands: Excerpta Medica, 1985:23-43.

9. McClearn GE, Rodgers DA. Differences in alcohol preference among inbred strains of mice. J Stud Alcohol. 1959; 20:691-695.

10. Mardones J. Experimentally induced changes in the free selection of ethanol. Int Rev Neurobiol. 1960; 2:41-76.

11. Eriksson K. Genetic selection for voluntary alcohol consumption in the albino rat. Science. 1968; 159:739-741.

12. Li T-K, Lumeng L, McBride WJ, Waller MB. Progress toward a voluntary oral consumption model of alcoholism. Drug Alcohol Depend. 1979; 4: 45-60.

13. Li T-K, Lumeng L, McBride WJ, Waller, MB. Indiana selection studies on alcohol-related behaviors. In: McClearn GE, Deitrich RA, Erwin VG, eds. Development of Animal Models as Pharmacogenetic Tools. National Institute on Alcohol Abuse and Alcoholism Research Monograph 6. Washington, DC: Supt of Docs, U.S. Government Printing Office.

14. Lumeng L, Doolittle DP, Li T-K. New duplicate lines of rats that differ in voluntary alcohol consumption. In: Abstracts of the Third Congress of the International Society for Biomedical Research on Alcoholism. Helsinki, Finland. Alcohol and Alcoholism, 1986; A37.

15. Lumeng L, Hawkins T, Li T-K. New strains of rats with alcohol preference and nonpreference. In: Thurman RG, Williamson JR, Drott HR, Chance B, eds. Alcohol and Aldehyde Metabolizing Systems. New York: Academic Press. 1977; III:537-544.

16. Waller MB, McBride WJ, Lumeng L, Li T-K. Induction of dependence on ethanol by free-choice drinking in alcohol-preferring rats. Pharmacol Biochem Behav. 1982; 16:501-507.

17. Lumeng L, Li T-K. The development of metabolic tolerance in the alcohol-preferring P rats: comparison of forced and free-choice drinking of ethanol. Pharmacol Biochem Behav. 1986; 25:1013-1020.

18. Murphy JM, Gatto GJ, Waller MB, McBride WJ, Lumeng L, Li T-K.

Effects of scheduled access on ethanol intake by the alcohol-preferring P line of rats. Alcohol. 1986; 3:331-336.

19. Waller MB, McBride WJ, Lumeng L, Li T-K. Effects of intravenous ethanol and of 4-methylpyrazole on alcohol drinking of alcohol-preferring rats. Pharmacol Biochem Behav. 1982; 17:763-768.

20. Tullis KB, Sargent WQ, Simpson JR, Beard JD. An animal model for the measurement of acute tolerance to ethanol. Life Sci. 1977; 20:875-882.

21. Gatto GJ, Murphy JM, McBride WJ, Lumeng L, Li T-K. Chronic ethanol tolerance through free-choice drinking in the P line of alcohol-preferring rats. Pharmacol Biochem Behav. 1987; 28:111-115.

22. Penn PE, McBride WJ, Lumeng L, Gaff TM, Li T-K. Neurochemical and operant behavioral studies of a strain of alcohol-preferring rats. Pharmacol Biochem Behav. 1978; 8:475-481.

23. Meisch RA. Ethanol self-administration: Infrahuman studies. In: Thompson T, Dews PB, eds. Advances in Behavioral Pharmacology. New York: Academic Press. 1977; 1:35-82.

24. Deutsch JA, Hardy WT. Ethanol tolerance in the rat measured by the untasted intake of alcohol. Behav Biol. 1976; 17:379-389.

25. Deutsch JA, Walton NY. A rat alcoholism model in a free-choice situation. Behav Biol. 1977; 19:349-360.

26. Waller MB, McBride WJ, Gatto GJ, Lumeng L, Li T-K. Intragastric ethanol self-administration by ethanol-preferring and -nonpreferring lines of rats. Science. 1984; 225:78-80.

27. Deutsch JA, Eisner A. Ethanol self-administration in the rat induced by forced drinking of ethanol. Behav Biol. 1977; 20:81-90.

28. Waller MB, Murphy JM, McBride WJ, Lumeng L, Li T-K. Effect of low dose ethanol on spontaneous motor activity in the alcohol-preferring (P) and -nonpreferring (NP) lines of rats. Pharmacol Biochem Behav. 1986; 24:617-625.

29. Morzorati S, Lamishaw B, Clemens J, Lumeng L, Li T-K. Alcoholism. Clin Exp Res. 1987; 11:207.

30. Waller MB, McBride WJ, Lumeng L, Li T-K. Initial sensitivity and acute tolerance to ethanol in the P and NP lines of rats. Pharmacol Biochem Behav. 1983; 19:683-686.

31. Gatto GJ, Murphy JM, McBride WJ, Lumeng L, Li T-K. Persistence of acute ethanol tolerance to a single dose of ethanol in the selectively bred alcohol-preferring P rats. Pharmacol Biochem Behav. 1987; 28:105-110.

32. Froehlich JC, Hostetler J, Lumeng L, Li T-K. Alcoholism. Clin Exp Res. 1987; 11:199.

33. Tabakoff B, Ritzman RF, Raju TS, Deitrich RA. Characterization of acute and chronic tolerance in mice selected for inherent differences in sensitivity to ethanol. Alcoholism. Clin Exp Res. 1980; 4:70-73.

34. Erwin VG, McClearn GE, Kuse AR. Interrelationships of alcohol consumption actions of alcohol and biochemical traits. Pharmacol Biochem Behav. 1980; 13(Suppl 1):297-302.

35. Nikander P, Pekkanen L. An inborn alcohol tolerance in alcohol-prefer-

ring rats. The lack of relationship between tolerance to ethanol and brain microsomal Na^+, K^+-ATPase activity. Psychopharmacology. 1977; 51:219-233.

36. Froehlich JC, Harts J, Lumeng L, Li T-K. Differences in ethanol-induced conditioned taste aversion between P and NP rats. Alcoholism. Clin Exp Res. 1986; 10:110.

37. Murphy JM, McBride WJ, Lumeng L, Li T-K. Regional brain levels of monoamines in alcohol-preferring and -nonpreferring lines of rats. Pharmacol Biochem Behav. 1982; 16:145-149.

38. Murphy JM, McBride WJ, Lumeng L, Li T-K. Alcohol preference and regional brain monoamine contents of N/Nih heterogeneous stock rats. Alcohol Drug Res. 1987; 7:33-39.

39. Murphy JM, McBride WJ, Lumeng L, Li T-K. Contents of monoamines in forebrain regions of the alcohol-preferring (P) and -nonpreferring (NP) lines of rats. Pharmacol Biochem Behav. 1987; 26:389-392.

40. Wong DT, Lumeng L, Threlkeld PG, Reid LR, Li T-K. J Neural Transmission. 1987 (in press).

41. Murphy JM, Waller MB, Gatto GJ, McBride WJ, Lumeng L, Li T-K. Monoamine uptake inhibitors attenuate ethanol intake in alcohol-preferring (P) rats. Alcohol. 1985; 2:349-352.

42. Waller MB, Murphy JM, McBride WJ, Lumeng L, Li T-K. Studies on the reinforcing properties of ethanol in alcohol-preferring (P) rats. Alcoholism. Clin Exp Res. 1985; 9:207.

43. Froehlich JC, Harts J, Lumeng L, Li T-K. Naloxone attenuation of voluntary alcohol consumption. In: Lindros KO, Ylikahri R, Kiianmaa K, eds. Advances in Biomedical Alcohol Research. Oxford: Pergamon Press. 1987; 333-338.

Characterization of Outward Currents in a Neurosecretory Cell Acutely Isolated from the Adult Rat

Luis G. Aguayo, PhD

SUMMARY. Hormonal release from neurosecretory cells appears to be regulated in part by ionic currents. Because ethanol was shown to alter the release of melatonin from the cultured pineal gland, the ionic currents present in pineal cells were characterized using the whole-cell patch clamp technique. The macroscopic ionic current observed in standard solutions was dominated by an outward current component. Study of this outward component in a solution without added external Ca^{2+} revealed the existence of two distinct outward currents. Depolarizing command voltages from a holding potential of -100 mV activated a fast outward current which reached a peak within 20 ms and completely decayed in about 150 ms. The second outward current isolated from a holding potential of -50 mV activated at potentials positive to -20 mV. In the presence of 2 mM external Ca^{2+} the I-V relationship did not display a region of negative slope conductance suggesting that Ca^{2+}-activated K^+ current did not contribute significantly to the outward current. A small Ca^{2+} inward current was observed when these two outward components were eliminated.

These results indicate that acutely dissociated pineal cells display two distinct K^+ outward currents: (i) a transient current similar to the A current (I_A); and (ii) a slowly activating, sustained current similar to the delayed rectifier (I_K). Thus, the characterization of ionic currents in the pineal cell is of importance because they may be a target for acute and chronic ethanol actions.

Luis G. Aguayo is affiliated with the Section of Electrophysiology, Laboratory of Physiologic and Pharmacologic Studies, Division of Intramural Clinical and Biological Research, National Institute on Alcohol Abuse and Alcoholism, 12501 Washington Avenue, Rockville, MD 20852.

Hormonal secretion from neurosecretory cells appears to be mediated in part by the activation of voltage-dependent membrane currents. The secretion of prolactin, melanocyte stimulating hormone, and growth hormone from pituitary cells can be either facilitated or depressed by dihydropyridine analogs.[1] Electrophysiological experiments suggest that these effects on hormonal secretion can be explained by the activation of a single type of Ca^{2+} channel.[2] For example, the inward current generated by this type of Ca^{2+} channel is activated by large depolarizing voltage steps and by BAY K8644, and it can be blocked by nifedipine. Recent studies have shown that ethanol alters the release of melatonin from the pineal gland.[3] Ethanol may exert this action by modification of membrane currents. Because it is currently unknown what types of membrane currents can be activated in these neurosecretory cells, this study was undertaken as a first step in characterizing the membrane response of individual rat pineal cells.

Single cells from the pineal gland were acutely separated with enzymatic techniques from male rats (200-300 g) kept under LD 12:12h with lights on from 6 a.m. to 6 p.m. Membrane responses of dispersed cells were studied using the whole-cell patch-clamp recording technique. Current pulses of variable amplitude produced a graded voltage response which was slightly enhanced by the addition of external Ca^{2+} or Ba^{2+}. In the presence of internal K^+, a rectification phenomena developed within 25 ms and it was blocked by internal $Cs+$. From a holding potential negative to -80 mV, the macroscopic ionic current observed in standard external (mM: 150 NaCl; 5.4 KCl; 2 $CaCl_2$; 1 $MgCl_2$; and 10 HEPES; pH 7.4) and internal solution (mM: 130 KCl; 1 $CaCl_2$; 2 $MgCl_2$; 10 HEPES; and 11 EGTA) was dominated by two outward current components. The cell input resistance measured at potentials between -60 and -120 mV was on the order of $2G\Omega$. A Ca^{2+} inward current, apparently similar to that seen in pituitary cells with an identical voltage protocol, was observed when the outward components were eliminated by the presence of internal Cs^+ in the patch pipette. In the presence of 10 mM external Ca^{2+}, this inward current activated slowly and it was sustained during a 60 ms pulse. From a holding potential of -50 mV, this current was activated at potentials positive to -40 mV and it peaked at about $+5$ mV. Increasing the holding potential to -80 mV shifted the threshold of activation of this current to -60 mV.

Two distinct outward currents were activated in a Ca^{2+}-free external solution. From a holding potential of -50 mV, depolarizing command voltages to -20 mV activated a sustained current. This current completely activated in 55 ms and displayed minimal inactivation within 400 ms. Tetraethylammonium (50 mM) blocked this response by over 80%. The second outward current isolated from a holding potential of -100 mV activated at potentials positive to -60 mV. This was a significantly faster current which reached a peak within 15 ms and completely decayed in about 150 ms. Application of 4 aminopyridine (5mM) and external Ca^{2+} (5mM) caused a reversible reduction of the current amplitude of this transient current. In the presence of 2 mM external Ca^{2+}, the I-V relationship for the delayed current did not display a region of negative slope conductance suggesting that Ca^{2+}-activated K^+ currents did not contribute significantly to the outward current. Cell-attached recordings revealed the presence of a high conductance outward single current. This channel was activated at depolarized patch potentials and it appeared to be a Ca^{2+}-dependent K^+ channel of the BK type.[4]

In conclusion, whole cell recordings indicate that acutely dissociated pineal cells display two distinct K^+ outward currents: (i) a slowly activating, sustained current similar to the delayed rectifier (I_K); and (ii) a transient current similar to the A current (I_A). Cell-attached experiments suggest the presence of a Ca^{2+} activated K^+ channel. Pineal cells did not display Na^+ currents and the inward component demonstrated in the absence of outward currents appeared to be a Ca^{2+} current. Thus, the characterization of ionic currents in adult pineal cells is of importance because they may be a possible target for acute and chronic ethanol actions.

REFERENCES

1. Cronin MJ, Anderson JM, Rogol AD, Koritnik DR, Thorner MO, Evans WS. Calcium channel agonist BAY K8644 enhances anterior pituitary secretion in rat and monkey. Am J Physiol 1985; 249:E326-E329.
2. Enyeart JJ, Sheu S-S, Hinkle PM. Dihydropyridine modulators of voltage-

sensitive Ca^2+ channels specifically regulate prolactin production by GH_4C_1 pituitary cells. J Biol Chem 1987; 262:3154-3159.

3. Moss HB, Tamarkin L, Majchrowicz E, Martin PR, Linnoila M. Pineal function during ethanol intoxication, dependence, and withdrawal. Life Sci 1986; 39:2209-2214.

4. Marty A, Neher E. Potassium channels in cultured bovine adrenal chromaffin cells. J Physiol 1985; 367:117-141.

Voltage-Clamp Models for the Study of Acute and Chronic Effects of Ethanol on Ionic Currents in Adult Mammalian Neurons

Stephen R. Ikeda, MD, PhD
Geoffrey G. Schofield, PhD
Forrest F. Weight, MD

SUMMARY. The aim of this study was to develop and characterize a model system in which the effects of ethanol on voltage- and agonist-gated ionic currents in adult mammalian neurons could be studied using voltage-clamp techniques. We have found that neurons enzymatically isolated from the peripheral (nodose and superior cervical ganglia) and central nervous system (pyramidal layer of the hippocampus) of the adult rat and guinea pig provide several advantages over conventional neuronal preparations (e.g., intact ganglia or brain slice). First, the isolated neurons, in conjunction with the patch clamp technique, allow high fidelity recordings of both macroscopic and single channel currents. Secondly, current- and voltage-clamp recordings have revealed that active and passive membrane properties, chemosensitivity, and ionic currents in the isolated neurons resemble those described from conventional preparations. Finally, we have developed an intracellular perfusion system which allows the convenient control of the intracellular milieu. This technique should be useful for the study of intracellular second messengers on ionic currents. Our results demonstrate that isolated adult mammalian neurons are ideally suited for the study of both the acute and chronic effects of ethanol on membrane excitability.

Stephen R. Ikeda, Geoffrey G. Schofield, and Forrest F. Weight are affiliated with the Section of Electrophysiology, Laboratory of Physiologic and Pharmacologic Studies, Division of Intramural Clinical and Biological Research, National Institute on Alcohol Abuse and Alcoholism, 12501 Washington Avenue, Rockville, MD 20852.

Reprint requests should be sent to Stephen R. Ikeda.

Most voltage-clamp studies of the effects of ethanol on membrane currents have been conducted on non-mammalian tissue. This study was undertaken to develop and characterize model systems suitable for the investigation of the effects of ethanol on voltage- and agonist-gated ionic currents in *adult mammalian neurons* using voltage-clamp techniques. We have found that neurons enzymatically isolated from the nodose[1,2] and superior cervical[3] ganglia of the adult rat and pyramidal layer of the hippocampus of the adult guinea pig[4] provide several advantages over conventional neuronal preparations (e.g., intact ganglia or brain slice). First, the isolated neurons, in conjunction with the patch-clamp technique, allow high fidelity recordings of both macroscopic and single channel currents. Furthermore, current- and voltage-clamp recordings have revealed that active and passive membrane properties, chemosensitivity, and ionic currents in the isolated neurons resemble those described from conventional preparations. Table 1 summarizes the various agonist- and voltage-gated currents we have found in these isolated neuron preparations. Since many of these currents have been implicated in

Table 1 Currents investigated in acutely dispersed adult mammalian neurons

Current	Nodose	SCG	Hippocampal
Inward Currents			
TTX-sensitive I_{Na}	+	+	+
TTX-resistant I_{Na}	+	-	?
Transient LVA I_{Ca}	+	-	+
Sustained HVA I_{Ca}	+	+	+
Outward Currents			
Ca-dependent I_K	+	+	+
Delayed rectifier	+	+	+
A-current	+	+	+
Agonist-gated Currents			
5-HT induced current	+	?	?
ACh induced current	?	+	?

the regulation of neuronal activity, these techniques will be useful for the elucidation of the mechanism(s) by which ethanol alters membrane excitability. Secondly, membrane currents can be studied in isolation by intra and extracellular ion substitution and pharmacological agents. Finally, we have modified the patch clamp technique to allow the convenient control of the intracellular milieu. This technique will be useful for the study of intracellular second messengers on ionic currents. Our results demonstrate that isolated adult mammalian neurons, in conjunction with the patch clamp technique, are ideally suited for the study of both the *acute* and *chronic* effects of ethanol on neuronal membrane excitability mechanisms.

REFERENCES

1. Ikeda SR, Schofield GG, Weight FF. Na^+ and Ca^{2+} currents of acutely isolated adult rat nodose ganglion cells. J Neurophysiol 1986; 55:527-539.

2. Ikeda SR, Schofield GG. Tetrodotoxin-resistant sodium current of rat nodose neurones: Monovalent cation selectivity and divalent cation block. J Physiol (Lond) 1987; 389: 255-270.

3. Ikeda SR, Schofield GG, Weight FF. Somatostatin blocks a calcium current in acutely isolated adult rat superior cervical ganglion neurons. Neurosci Lett 1987; 81:123-128.

4. Kay AR, Wong RKS. Isolation of neurons suitable for patch-clamping from adult mammalian central nervous systems. J Neurosci Meth 1986; 16:227-238.

Ethanol's Effects
on Neurotransmitter Release
and Intracellular Free Calcium
in PC12 Cells

C. S. Rabe, PhD
F. F. Weight, MD

SUMMARY. The effect of ethanol on muscarine-stimulated release of [³H]NE was studied using the rat pheochromocytoma cell line, PC12. At concentrations of 25 mM and above, ethanol produced a dose dependent inhibition of muscarine-stimulated release of [³H]NE. The inhibition of muscarine-stimulated transmitter release occurred in the absence of any effect of ethanol on [³H]NE uptake, metabolism or on muscarinic binding to the cells. However, ethanol produced an inhibition of muscarine-stimulated elevation of intracellular free Ca^{2+} which corresponded with the inhibition of transmitter release. At concentrations greater than 100 mM, ethanol produced both a stimulation of the release of [³H]NE as well as an increase in intracellular free Ca^{2+}. The increase in basal transmitter release and intracellular free Ca^{2+} occurred independent of the inhibition by ethanol of muscarine-stimulated elevation of intracellular free Ca^{2+} or transmitter secretion. These results demonstrate the relationship of the effects of ethanol on cellular free Ca^{2+} and neurotransmitter release.

Acute ethanol intoxication is believed to be due to disruption of normal patterns of neurotransmission. However, it is unknown precisely how ethanol disrupts transmitter release. The rat pheochro-

C. S. Rabe and F. F. Weight are affiliated with the Laboratory of Physiologic and Pharmacologic Studies, National Institute on Alcohol Abuse and Alcoholism, 12501 Washington Avenue, Rockville, MD 20852.
Reprint requests should be sent to C. S. Rabe.

mocytoma cell line, PC12, secretes catecholamines in response to a variety of stimuli in a manner similar to sympathetic neurons.[1] By utilizing PC12 cells as a model for neurosecretion, it is possible to study the effects of ethanol on secretion as well as the processes which underlie secretion.

Recently, we have described muscarine-evoked secretion of [3H]norepinephrine ([3H]NE) from these cells.[2] In the presence of concentrations of ethanol as low as 25 mM, muscarine-stimulated secretion of [3H]NE is rapidly and reversibly inhibited. Table 1 shows the effect of increasing concentrations of ethanol on the [3H]NE released in response to 100 μM muscarine. The inhibition of muscarine-evoked transmitter release occurred in the absence of any effect of ethanol on [3H]NE uptake or metabolism. In addition,

Table 1

Effect of Ethanol on Muscarine-Stimulated [3H]NE Release and

Elevation of Intracellular Free Ca^{2+}

Ethanol (mM)	[3H]NE Released (% of Control)	Net Increase in Intracelluar Free Ca^{2+} (% of Control)
10	92.8 ± 2.6	N.D.
25	86.1 ± 2.7*	N.D.
50	85.4 ± 1.4*	N.D.
100	74.3 ± 2.6*	73.2 ± 5.8*
200	61.3 ± 2.3*	N.D.
400	36.9 ± 3.2*	50.8 ± 6.3*

The release of [3H]NE was determined as described previously[2]. The net increase in intracellular free Ca^{2+} was determined using Quin 2 as described previously[2]. * $p < 0.01$ as determined using ANOVA, n=7-12. N.D.= not done.

ethanol had no effect on muscarinic binding to the cells, indicating that the inhibition of secretion occurred at a step in the stimulus-secretion coupling process subsequent to agonist binding.

Elevation of intracellular free Ca^{2+} is known to play an important role in the stimulation of transmitter release and we previously have shown that the release of [^{3}H]NE evoked by muscarine correlates well with the ability of muscarine to elevate intracellular free Ca^{2+}.[2] As seen in Table 1, ethanol inhibits muscarine-stimulated transmitter release and muscarine-stimulated (10 μM) elevation of intracellular free Ca^{2+} to a similar degree. Since muscarine-stimulated increases in intracellular free Ca^{2+} appear to result from mobilization of Ca^{2+} from intracellular stores,[2] these results suggest that ethanol may inhibit transmitter release by limiting the ability of muscarine to mobilize intracellular stores of Ca^{2+}.

At concentrations of ethanol of 100 mM or less, ethanol has no effect on the basal rate of transmitter release. However, at concentrations greater than 100 mM, ethanol causes elevation of the basal rate of transmitter release. Ethanol (400 mM) causes approximately a 20% increase in the basal rate of [^{3}H]NE release. This increase in [^{3}H]NE release was accompanied by an elevation of the basal level of intracellular free Ca^{2+}. For example 400 mM ethanol raises the level of intracellular free Ca^{2+} from 114 ± 2 nM to 149 ± 4 nM (mean $\pm$ S.E.M., $n = 7$). The increase in basal transmitter release and intracellular free Ca^{2+} occurred independently of the inhibition by ethanol of muscarine-stimulated elevation of intracellular free Ca^{2+} or transmitter secretion. These results demonstrate the close relationship of the effects of ethanol on intracellular free Ca^{2+} and neurotransmitter release.

REFERENCES

1. Greene L.A. and Tischler, A.S. PC12 pheochromocytoma cultures in neurobiological research. Adv. Cell. Neurobiol. 1982; 3: 373-414.

2. Rabe, C.S., DeLorme, E. and Weight, F.F. Muscarine stimulated neurotransmitter release from PC12 cells. J. Pharmacol. Exp. Ther. 1987; 243: 534-541.

Effects of Chronic Ethanol Ingestion on Mouse Brain β-Adrenergic Receptors (BAR) and Adenylate Cyclase

P. Valverius, MD
P. L. Hoffman, PhD
B. Tabakoff, PhD

SUMMARY. Previous work showed that chronic ethanol ingestion by C57BL mice resulted in reduced stimulation of cerebral cortical adenylate cyclase (AC) activity by isoproterenol (ISO) and guanine nucleotides (GN). To investigate the mechanism of this change we have assessed the effect of chronic ethanol ingestion on agonist and antagonist binding to BAR in cerebral cortex (mainly β1-AR) and cerebellum (mainly β2-AR). C57BL mice were fed ethanol in a liquid diet for seven days and were withdrawn for various intervals. Agonist (ISO) binding data were best fit by a two-site model (high and low affinity states) in cortical membranes of control mice. GN induced conversion to a one site model (low affinity state). At the time of withdrawal, ISO binding data in cortical membranes were best fit by a one-site model even in the absence of GN. Antagonist binding was not affected. These results resemble those seen after heterologous desensitization, indicating "uncoupling" of receptor and AC. Control cerebellar ISO binding data were similar to cortical data. Chronic ethanol ingestion, however, did not produce data fit by a one site model in cerebellum. The affinity for ISO of the high affinity state of the BAR was significantly decreased at the time of withdrawal. ISO-stimulated AC-activity in cerebellar membranes

P. Valverius, P. L. Hoffman, and B. Tabakoff are affiliated with the Division of Intramural Clinical and Biological Research, National Institute on Alcohol Abuse and Alcoholism, 12501 Washington Avenue, Rockville, MD 20852.

P. Valverius is a Fogarty Research Fellow. Reprint requests should be sent to him.

This research was supported in part by the Swedish Medical Research Council, Contract No. K-85-25R7296, and by the Banbury Foundation.

was not affected by chronic ethanol ingestion, indicating that, in contrast to cerebral cortex, the cerebellar BAR was not uncoupled from AC.

Stimulation of adenylate cyclase (AC) activity requires the presence of at least two other membrane-bound proteins: a receptor and a guanine nucleotide binding protein (Gs).[1] Previous work has shown that chronic ingestion of ethanol by C57BL mice resulted in reduced stimulation of cerebral cortical AC activity by guanine nucleotides (Gpp(NH)p) and isoproterenol (ISO).[2] Furthermore, it has been reported that chronic ethanol ingestion in mice led to the disappearance of the high-affinity (HA) agonist (ISO) binding site of the cerebral cortical beta-adrenergic receptor and to a small, but significant decrease in the total number of ISO binding sites at the time of ethanol withdrawal.[3] These changes were no longer apparent by 72 hours after withdrawal.[3] To investigate the specificity of these responses to ethanol we have evaluated the effect of chronic ethanol ingestion on antagonist (ICYP) and agonist (ISO) binding to BAR, and on AC stimulation by Gpp(NH)p and ISO in membrane preparations from C57BL mouse cerebellum.

Antagonist binding: Chronic ethanol ingestion, leading to functional tolerance and physical dependence, significantly decreased the number of cerebellar ICYP binding sites, while the affinity for ICYP was not affected. ICYP binding returned to the control level within 72 hours after ethanol withdrawal.

Agonist binding: In cerebellar membranes, the proportion of high- and low-affinity ISO binding forms of BAR was not altered after chronic ethanol ingestion. Although the total number of ISO-binding sites was lowered, this change did not reach statistical significance. The affinity for ISO of the HA ISO binding form of the receptor was significantly decreased.

AC activity: Chronic ingestion of ethanol did not affect basal AC activity, maximal responses to Gpp(NH)p or ISO or the EC50 for ISO stimulation of AC in cerebellar membrane preparations.

Discussion: The earlier finding that the HA agonist binding form of the BAR in cerebral cortical membranes is undetectable after chronic ethanol ingestion suggested that the cortical BAR is "uncoupled" from AC at the time of ethanol withdrawal.[3] These results are consistent with the previous study showing reduced stimulation of cerebral cortical AC by Gpp(NH)p and ISO at the time of ethanol withdrawal.[2] The changes are similar to those occurring during heterologous desensitization, in which the amount of the HA agonist binding form of the BAR is lowered,[1] possibly due to a deficiency in Gs.

In contrast, the data obtained with cerebellar membranes do not support the postulate that the BAR is uncoupled from AC. The decreased affinity for ISO and the slightly decreased number of the cerebellar HA agonist binding sites did not appear to affect the functional response to agonist, i.e., activation of AC.

The difference in the effect of chronic ethanol ingestion on cerebral cortical and cerebellar BAR-coupled AC could be related to the different populations of BAR in these regions. The cerebral cortical beta-1 AR[4] have been suggested to be neuronal (i.e., within the blood-brain-barrier, BBB) while the cerebellar beta-2 AR[4] are suggested to be non-neuronal (e.g., vascular, outside the BBB), and thus subject to greater peripheral influences from, for example, circulating catecholamines, as well as ethanol.

REFERENCES

1. Sibley, D.R., R.J. Lefkowitz. Molecular mechanisms of receptor desensitization using the beta-adrenergic receptor-coupled adenylate cyclase system as a model. Nature 1985, 317: 214-229.

2. Saito, T., J.M. Lee, P.L. Hoffman, B. Tabakoff. Effects of chronic ethanol treatment on the beta-adrenergic receptor-coupled adenylate cyclase system in mouse cerebral cortex. J. Neurochem. 1987, 48: 1817-1822.

3. Valverius, P., P.L. Hoffman, B. Tabakoff. Effect of ethanol on mouse cerebral cortical beta-adrenergic receptors. Mol. Pharmacol. 1987, 32: 217-224.

4. Severson, J.A., R.N. Pittman, J. Gal, P.B. Molinoff, C.E. Finch. Genetic influence on the regulation of beta-adrenergic receptors in mice. J. Pharmacol. Exp. Ther. 1985, 236: 24-29.

Cholera Toxin-Induced ADP-Ribosylation of a 46kDa Protein Is Decreased in Brains of Ethanol-Fed Mice

P. T. Nhamburo, PhD
P. L. Hoffman, PhD
B. Tabakoff, PhD

SUMMARY. The acute *in vitro* effects of ethanol on cerebral cortical adenylate cyclase activity and beta-adrenergic receptor characteristics suggested a site of action of ethanol at G_s, the stimulatory guanine nucleotide binding protein. After chronic ethanol ingestion, the beta-adrenergic receptor appeared to be uncoupled (i.e., the form of the receptor with high affinity for agonist was undetectable), and stimulation of adenylate cyclase activity by isoproterenol or guanine nucleotides was reduced, suggesting an alteration in the properties of G_s. To further characterize this change, cholera and pertussis toxin-mediated ^{32}P-ADP-ribosylation of mouse cortical membranes was assessed in mice that had chronically ingested ethanol in a liquid diet. ^{32}P-labeled proteins were separated by SDS-PAGE and quantitated by autoradiography. There was a selective 30-50% decrease in cholera toxin-induced labeling of 46kDa protein band in membranes of ethanol-fed mice, with no apparent change in pertussis toxin-induced labeling. The 46kDa protein has a molecular weight similar to that of the alpha subunit of G_s, suggesting a reduced amount of this protein or a change in its characteristics as a substrate for cholera toxin-induced ADP-ribosylation in cortical membranes of ethanol-fed mice.

P. T. Nhamburo, P. L. Hoffman, and B. Tabakoff are affiliated with the Division of Intramural Clinical and Biological Research, National Institute on Alcohol Abuse and Alcoholism, 12501 Washington Avenue, Rockville, MD 20852. This research supported in part by the Banbury Foundation.

Reprint requests should be sent to P. L. Hoffman.

Three classes of protein components have been implicated in the regulation of hormone-sensitive adenylate cyclase (AC) systems: hormone receptor, guanine nucleotide binding proteins (G-proteins) and the catalytic unit (C) of AC.[1] Previous data from our laboratory supported the postulate that a decrease in the function or amount of G_s (stimulatory G-protein) is a factor in the decrease in Gpp(NH)p and isoproterenol (ISO) stimulation of AC,[2] and in the changes in β-adrenergic receptor properties,[3] that are observed in cerebral cortical membranes of mice fed ethanol chronically. Cholera toxin, in the presence of NAD^+, ADP-ribosylates a site on G_s, while pertussis toxin catalyzes the ADP-ribosylation of G_i (the inhibitory guanine nucleotide binding protein) and G_o.[4]

We have quantitated the levels of these G-proteins in cerebral cortex of mice that have chronically ingested ethanol by measuring toxin-catalyzed ^{32}P-ADP-ribosylation of cortical proteins, separated by SDS-polyacrylamide gel electrophoresis (PAGE).

C57BL mice were fed ethanol in a liquid diet, or control liquid diet, for seven days.[5] Cerebral cortical membranes were incubated with 0.1mM [α-^{32}P] NAD^+ for 60 min at 30°C in the presence or absence of activated toxin (either 50 μg/ml cholera toxin or 2.5 μg/ml pertussis toxin). [^{32}P]-labeled proteins were separated by SDS-PAGE and quantitated by autoradiography. Under the conditions used, ADP-ribosylation was sensitive to changes in the concentration of the toxin substrates.

Cholera toxin mediated the incorporation of radioactivity into several membrane proteins. A 46 kilodalton (kDa) protein, which has the same molecular weight as the alpha subunit of G_s ($α_s$), constituted a major substrate of the toxin. On the other hand, pertussis toxin ADP-ribosylated a single protein band (39 kDa). The patterns of membrane proteins ADP-ribosylated by either cholera or pertussis toxin in membranes of ethanol-fed mice that were sacrificed at the time of withdrawal were not significantly different from those in naive (chow-fed) mice or mice fed control liquid diet. However, in the mice fed ethanol chronically there was a significant decrease (approximately 40 percent) in the amount of radioactivity incorporated into the 46 kDa protein. The decrease in labeling was specific for this protein. That is, no significant changes were observed in the incorporation of radioactivity by other membrane-bound proteins that were ADP-ribosylated in the presence of either cholera or pertussis toxin.

The decrease in the amount of radioactivity incorporated into the 46 kDa protein, which has properties similar to the alpha subunit of G_s (i.e., it is a substrate of cholera toxin and has a molecular weight similar to α_s), suggests that there may be a decrease in the amount of this protein, or a change in its availability for ribosylation, in cerebral cortical membranes of ethanol-fed mice.

REFERENCES

1. Rodbell, M. Nature 1980, *284*: 17-22.
2. Saito, T., Lee, J.M., Hoffman, P.L., Tabakoff, B. J. Neurochem. 1987, *48*: 1817-1822.
3. Valverius, P., Hoffman, P.L., Tabakoff B. Mol. Pharmacol. 1987, *32*: 217-222.
4. Gilman, A.G. Cell 1984, *36*: 577-579.
5. Ritzmann, R.F., Tabakoff, B. J. Pharmacol. Exptl. Ther. 1976, *199*: 158-170.

Measuring the Serotonin Uptake Site Using [3H]Paroxetine — A New Serotonin Uptake Inhibitor

Christoph H. Gleiter, MD
David J. Nutt, MD, PhD

SUMMARY. Serotonin is an important neurotransmitter that may be involved in ethanol preference and dependence. It is possible to label the serotonin uptake site in brain using the tricyclic antidepressant imipramine, but this also binds to other sites. We have used the new high-affinity uptake blocker paroxetine to define binding to this site and report it to have advantages over imipramine as a ligand.

Serotonin (5-HT) is a neurotransmitter that may be involved in ethanol preference and dependence. Data from animal experiments show that 5-HT seems to be involved in alcohol appetite, preference and tolerance.[1] Some abstinent alcoholics show a reduced 5-HT function (indicated by low CSF 5-HIAA). These results suggest a low CSF 5-HIAA concentration to be an inherited trait that may predispose to alcoholism.[2] The platelet 5-HT uptake site is regarded as a possible marker of certain brain 5-HT functions.[1,3] This binding site is usually labeled with [3H]imipramine although this probably labels a different site from the 5-HT transporter complex.[4] Furthermore imipramine binds to other receptors, such as those for histamine, acetylcholine and norepinephrine.[5] Paroxetine is a new potent and selective inhibitor of 5-HT uptake and is chemically different

Christoph H. Gleiter and David J. Nutt are affiliated with the Laboratory of Clinical Studies, Division of Intramural Clinical and Biological Research, National Institute on Alcohol Abuse and Alcoholism, NIH Clinical Center, Bldg. 10, Rm. 3B19, Bethesda, MD 20892.

Reprint requests should be sent to Christoph H. Gleiter.

from tricyclic antidepressants. Recently it has been characterized as a highly selective ligand for the 5-HT uptake site in rat brain.[6] Additional evidence suggests that human platelets have an identical binding site for [3H]paroxetine.[3]

As a first application of [3H]paroxetine binding we studied the effects of repeated electroshock (ECS). ECS treatment is considered to be a very effective therapy for severe depression. Recent studies have shown that it has marked effects on 5-HT function[7] and receptors in animals.[8] However, there exists no information about the effects of ECS on the 5-HT uptake site. Reports on the effect of chronic ECS on the [3H]imipramine binding site are conflicting.[8,9,10] Male Sprague-Dawley rats were treated with ECS once-daily over 10 days (80 mA, 0.5 s) via earclip electrodes and without anaesthesia. Twenty-four hours after the last treatment the animals were decapitated and the brains dissected. Equilibrium saturation studies with [3H]paroxetine were carried out as described by Habert.[6] Additionally single point binding was studied using [3H]imipramine at a concentration of 5 nM.[5] Results are given in Table 1.

In a further experiment [3H]paroxetine binding in cortex of genetically obese mice (C57BL/6J ob/ob), their lean littermates (C57BL/6J + /?) and NIH Swiss mice was measured (Table 2). The homozygous obese mouse has been reported to have elevated cerebral 5-HT levels.[11]

The present studies show that [3H]paroxetine binding is not af-

TABLE 1. Densities of binding sites (Bmax, fmol/mg protein) and equilibrium dissociation constants (Kd, nM) for [3H]paroxetine (n = 9), plus [3H]imipramine (n = 9) single point binding (5 nM; fmol/mg protein) after repeated ECS. There was no statistically significant difference for all parameters (mean ± SEM).

| | [3H] Paroxetine | | [3H] Imipramine |
	Bmax	Kd	
ECS	597 ± 36.5	0.06 ± 0.003	285 ± 16
Controls	628 ± 28.4	0.05 ± 0.003	283 ± 16

TABLE 2. Bmax and Kd in cortex membrane preparations of 100 day old genetically obese mice (ob/ob), their lean littermates (+/?), and NIH Swiss mice. Values represent the mean ± SEM of 3 cortex membrane preparations, each com-
prising cortices of 5 mice. There was no statistically significant difference for
either parameter.

	Bmax (fmol/mg protein)	Kd (nM)
ob/ob	649 ± 88.5	0.06 ± 0.0003
+/?	656 ± 9.1	0.05 ± 0.003
NIH Swiss	657 ± 51.1	0.07 ± 0.02

fected by repeated ECS. Secondly it is not altered in ob/ob mice in
spite of higher 5-HT levels compared with lean littermates and NIH
Swiss mice. In both experiments values of Bmax and Kd were not
different from controls and similar to previously reported values.[3,6]
The unchanged binding of [3H]imipramine after repeated ECS con-
firms a report by Stockmeier and Kellar.[8]

Briley proposed a model for the 5-HT uptake complex where
[3H]imipramine binds to a high affinity site which is closely related, yet not identical with the uptake mechanism for 5-HT and
may modulate this uptake noncompetitively via a sodium-depen-
dent allosteric interaction.[4] Tricyclic antidepressants can be expected to act at this site, whereas the non-tricyclic 5-HT uptake
inhibitors (e.g., paroxetine, fluoxetine) may act at the 5-HT uptake
site. The multiple receptor interactions and heterogeneity of
[3H]imipramine binding might explain the inconsistent results after
ECS.[8,9,10] The presence of additional non-serotonergic [3H]imip-
ramine binding sites could explain why paroxetine has been reported to inhibit [3H]imipramine binding to cortical membranes in a
complex fashion.[6]

A methodological advantage is that [3H]paroxetine assays can be
carried out at room temperature or even at body temperature.[6]
[3H]Imipramine has to be used at 0° C due to unfavourable binding
kinetics.[6] A comparison between [3H]imipramine binding in brain

and platelets revealed a tenfold difference in the Kd for [3H]imipramine whereas [3H]paroxetine binding was similar in both tissues.[3] This may indicate an identical binding site in neuronal and platelet membranes for [3H]paroxetine but not for [3H]imipramine. Therefore studies of the 5-HT uptake site in depressed patients or alcoholics might better be carried out using [3H]paroxetine than [3H]imipramine.

In conclusion [3H]paroxetine may be an appropriate ligand for the examination of the 5-HT uptake site due to its specific and potent inhibition of 5-HT uptake and its binding characteristics.

REFERENCES

1. Nutt D, Glue P. Monoamines and alcohol. Brit J Addiction. 1986, 81: 327-358.

2. Roy A, Virkunnen M, Linnoila M. Reduced central serotonin turnover in a subgroup of alcoholics? Prog Neuro-Psychopharmacol & Biol Psychiat. 1987, 11: 173-177.

3. Mellerup ET, Plenge P. High affinity binding of [3H]paroxetine and [3H]imipramine to rat neuronal membranes. Psychopharmacology. 1986, 89: 436-9.

4. Briley M. Imipramine binding: Its relationship with serotonin uptake and depression. In: Green AR, ed. Neuropharmacology of serotonin. Oxford: Oxford University Press. 1986: 50-78.

5. Snyder SH. Imipramine binding sites: Antidepressant actions at neurotransmitter receptors. In: Usdin E, Bunnney WE, Davis JM, eds. Neuroreceptors—basic and clinical aspects. Chichester and New York: J.Wiley. 1981: 154-164.

6. Habert E, Graham D, Tahraoui L, Claustre Y, Langer SZ. Characterization of [3H]paroxetine binding to rat cortical membranes. Europ J Pharmacol. 1985, 118: 107-114.

7. Green AR, Nutt DJ. Psychopharmacology of repeated seizures: Possible relevance to the mechanism of action of electroconvulsive therapy (ECT). In: Iversen LL, Iversen SD, Snyder SH, eds. Handbook of Psychopharmacology, vol 19. New directions in behavioral pharmacology. New York: Plenum Press. 1987: 375-408.

8. Stockmeier CA, Kellar KJ. In vivo regulation of the serotonin-2 receptor in rat brain. Life Sci. 1986, 38: 117-127.

9. Barkin AI. Interactions of drugs and electroshock treatment on cerebral monoaminergic systems. In: Malitz S, Sackeim H, eds. Electroconvulsive ther-

apy: clinical and basic research issues. Ann New York Acad Sci. 1986, 462: 147-162.

10. Langer SZ, Zarifian E, Briley M, Raisman R, Sechter D. High affinity binding of [3H]imipramine in brain and platelets and its relevance to the biochemistry of affective disorders. Life Sci. 1981, 20: 211-220.

11. Garthwaite TL, Kalkhoff RK, Guansing AR, Hagen TC, Menahan LA. Plasma free tryptophan, brain serotonin and endocrine profile of the genetically obese hyperglycemic mouse at 4-5 months of age. Endocrinology. 1979, 106: 1178-1182.

Interactions of 5HT
Reuptake Inhibitors
and Ethanol in Tests
of Exploration and Anxiety

M. J. Durcan, PhD
R. G. Lister, PhD
M. J. Eckardt, PhD
M. Linnoila, MD, PhD

SUMMARY. Treatment with 5HT reuptake inhibitors has been shown to attenuate ethanol consumption in both animals and humans. These experiments investigate in mice the interactions of the 5HT reuptake inhibitors fluoxetine, citalopram and fluvoxamine and the NA uptake inhibitor desipramine with ethanol in the holeboard test and the elevated plusmaze test of anxiety. Ethanol (2.4g/kg) increased activity both in the holeboard and on the plusmaze, decreased both the number and duration of head-dips in the holeboard, and increased both the percentage time and percentage entries on to the open-arm of the plusmaze (reflecting its anxiolytic properties). On their own, the selective 5HT uptake inhibitors fluoxetine, fluvoxamine, and citalopram and the NA uptake inhibitor desipramine (10-20mg/kg) did not significantly alter any of the behavioral measures. The only consistent interaction was seen with fluoxetine which reduced ethanol's anxiolytic effects at the 20mg/kg dose without altering ethanol's effects on exploration or locomotion. The results suggest that the attenuation of ethanol's anxiolytic properties by fluoxetine may not be serotonin related since other 5HT reuptake inhibitors did not show this effect at the doses used.

The authors are affiliated with the Laboratory of Clinical Studies, Division of Intramural Clinical and Biological Research, National Institute on Alcohol Abuse and Alcoholism, NIH Clinical Center, Bldg. 10, Rm. 3C218, Bethesda, MD 20892.

Reprint requests should be sent to M. J. Durcan.

INTRODUCTION

Treatment with 5HT uptake inhibitors has been shown to attenuate ethanol consumption in both animals[1] and humans,[2] however there is little behavioral evidence to account for this effect. In the following experiments the behavioral actions of the specific 5HT uptake inhibitor fluoxetine[3] and its interactions with ethanol were explored in mice.

The experiments reported here investigate the effects of pretreatment with fluoxetine on ethanol-induced changes of performance in both the holeboard test of exploration and locomotor activity[4] and the plusmaze test of anxiety.[5] The ethanol interactions of other 5HT uptake inhibitors, fluvoxamine and citalopram, and the selective noradrenaline uptake inhibitor desipramine were also investigated.

MATERIALS AND METHODS

Holeboard Testing

The holeboard apparatus consisted of a Plexiglas box (40 × 40 × 40cm) with four equally spaced holes (3cm in diameter) in the floor. Infra-red photocells in the walls and directly beneath each hole provided automated measures of motor activity and directed exploration (head-dipping). The holeboard testing, which took place in a dimly lit room, involved placing a mouse in the centre of the floor and allowing it to explore the box for 5 min.

Plusmaze Testing

The plusmaze apparatus was made of black Plexiglas and consisted of two opposite facing open arms (30 × 5cm) and two opposite facing closed arms (30 × 5cm) with a 5 × 5cm central area, the closed arms having clear Plexiglas walls 15cm high which were open at the ends: the whole apparatus was mounted on a base which raised it 38.5cm above the floor. The testing involved placing a mouse in the middle of the maze facing an open arm and allowing it to explore for 5 min.

The measures obtained from the plusmaze are: (1) Percentage of total arm-entries which were made onto the open arm; (2) The time spent on the open arm as a percentage of the total time spent on both the open and closed arms; and (3) The total number of arm entries.

EXPERIMENT 1

Six groups of NIH Swiss mice (N = 7-10) were administered 0, 10, or 20mg/kg fluoxetine i.p. (at a volume of 1 ml/100g) 90 min prior to testing followed by an i.p. injection of either 0 or 2.4g/kg ethanol in distilled water vehicle (at a volume of 2ml/100g) 30 min prior to testing in the holeboard followed by the plusmaze test.

Results

Ethanol significantly increased locomotor activity, as demonstrated both by total number of arm-entries on the plusmaze and holeboard motor activity. It decreased exploratory behavior (both number and duration of head-dips). Ethanol's anxiolytic properties were demonstrated by increases in the percentage entries and percentage time spent on the open-arm of the plusmaze. Fluoxetine alone had no effect on any of the locomotor, exploratory or anxiety measures.

There were interactions between fluoxetine and ethanol for the anxiety measures and comparison of the fluoxetine pretreated ethanol groups with the ethanol alone group showed significantly lowered scores for both percentage of entries and percentage of time spent on the open arms of the plusmaze at the 20mg/kg dose. There were no interactions between fluoxetine and ethanol on any other measures.

EXPERIMENT 2

In this study the selective 5HT uptake inhibitors fluvoxamine and citalopram and the noradrenaline uptake inhibitor desipramine were investigated using the same design and doses as experiment 1.

Results

The results of this experiment demonstrate the same ethanol effects on the locomotor, exploratory and anxiety measures observed in experiment 1. All three drugs showed no intrinsic effects on locomotor activity, directed exploration or anxiety. Neither of the 5HT uptake inhibitors showed any significant interaction with the anxiolytic properties of ethanol. Both doses of citalopram did however significantly increase the locomotor stimulant effects of ethanol seen in the holeboard and the 20mg/kg dose of fluvoxamine enhanced the ethanol-induced increase in total plusmaze arm-entries. No significant interactions were seen between desipramine and ethanol.

A summary of the effects of drugs used in both experiment 1 and experiment 2 on ethanol-induced behavioral changes is presented in Table 1.

CONCLUSIONS

(1) Fluoxetine has no intrinsic effects on locomotor activity, exploratory behavior or anxiety in the holeboard and plusmaze tests in mice.

TABLE 1: The effects of fluoxetine, fluvoxamine, citalopram ,and desipramine pretreatment (10-20mg/kg i.p.) on ethanol-induced (2.4g/kg i.p.) behavioral changes in the plusmaze and holeboard tests.

- attenuation of effects seen at 20mg/kg; + potentiation of effect seen at 20mg/gl; ++ potentiation of effect seen at 10 & 20 mg/kg.

	FLUOXETINE	FLUVOXAMINE	CITALOPRAM	DESIPRAMINE
ANXIOLYTIC EFFECT (PLUSMAZE)	-	none	none	none
INCREASED ARM-ENTRIES (PLUSMAZE)	none	+	none	none
REDUCTION OF EXPLORATION (HOLEBOARD HEAD-DIPPING)	none	none	none	none
INCREASED LOCOMOTOR ACTIVITY (HOLEBOARD)	none	none	++	none

(2) Fluoxetine (20mg/kg) selectively attenuates the anxiolytic properties of ethanol (as measured by the plusmaze test) without interacting with any of the other ethanol-induced behavioral changes.

(3) Fluoxetine's interaction with the anxiolytic properties of ethanol would not appear to be directly related to 5HT uptake inhibition per se since this effect is not seen with other selective 5HT uptake inhibitors (citalopram and fluoxamine), nor would it appear to be caused by noradrenaline uptake inhibition because no similar effect was seen after desipramine.

REFERENCES

1. Amit Z, Sutherland A, Gill K, Ogren SO. Zimeldine: A review of its effects on ethanol consumption. Neurosci and Biobehav Rev 1984; 8:35-53.

2. Naranjo CA, Sellars ED, Roach CA, Woodley DV, Sanchez-Craig M, Sykora K. Zimelidine-induced variations in alcohol intake by nondepressed heavy drinkers. Clin Pharmacol Ther 1985; 35:374-81.

3. Wong DT, Bymaster FP, Horng JS, Molloy BB. A new selective inhibitor for uptake of serotonin into synaptosomes of rat brain: 3-(p-trifluoromethyl); phenoxy-N-methyl-phenylpropylamine. J. Pharmacol Exp Ther 1975; 193: 804-11.

4. File SE, Wardill AG. Validity of head-dipping as a measure of exploration in a modified holeboard. Psychopharmacology 1975; 44:53-59.

5. Handley SL, Mithani S. Effects of alpha-adrenoceptor agonists and antagonists in a maze-exploration model of fear-motivated behavior. Nauyn-Schmied Arc Pharmacol 1984; 327:1-5.

RO 15-4513 and Its Interaction with Ethanol

Richard G. Lister, PhD
David J. Nutt, MD, PhD

SUMMARY. It has recently been claimed that RO 15-4513 selectively opposes some of the behavioral actions of ethanol. Our studies on the intrinsic effects of this compound have shown it to be proconvulsant and to reduce exploratory behavior in mice. In these respects RO 15-4513 resembles a benzodiazepine receptor partial inverse agonist. Such intrinsic actions may well explain its alcohol-antagonizing properties, and argue against its potential in humans. In addition to partially reversing the effects of ethanol, RO 15-4513 also partially reverses the behavioral effect of a barbiturate and completely reverses the effects of a benzodiazepine.

Over the last few years several groups have reported that the imidazodiazepine RO 15-4513 is capable of antagonising some of the electrophysiological and behavioral effects of ethanol.[1-3] These effects seemed to be mediated via the benzodiazepine receptor since they were reversed by the benzodiazepine receptor antagonist RO 15-1788.[1,3] It has been suggested these findings might lead to the development of a clinically effective ethanol antagonist. We now review the more recent literature, including our own studies which cast some doubt on this possibility.

The first question to be addressed is whether RO 15-4513 is a selective antagonist of ethanol, i.e., does RO 15-4513 only oppose

Richard G. Lister and David J. Nutt are affiliated with the Laboratory of Clinical Studies, Division of Intramural Clinical and Biological Research, National Institute on Alcohol Abuse and Alcoholism, NIH Clinical Center, Bldg. 10, Rm 3C218, Bethesda, MD 20892.
Reprint requests should be sent to Richard G. Lister.

the effects of ethanol, and not those of other CNS depressants. The *in vitro* work of Suzdak et al.[3] suggests that RO 15-4513 is particularly selective in reversing ethanol's stimulatory effect on GABA-mediated 36-chloride flux in synaptoneurosomal preparations, having no effect on barbiturate or GABA mediated stimulation. The same paper also showed, in a conflict paradigm, RO 15-4513 reversing the anticonflict effects of ethanol but not those of pentobarbital. In contrast to these findings, Britton et al.[4] found that RO 15-4513 reversed the effects of both ethanol and pentobarbital in their conflict test. Our studies in mice using both a seizure threshold paradigm[5] and a holeboard test of exploratory behavior[6] have found RO 15-4513 to interact with ethanol and sodium pentobarbital in a similar manner. The group at Hoffmann-La Roche has shown that RO 15-4513 reversed the effect of both ethanol and phenobarbitone in the horizontal wire test in mice.[1] However, it reversed the effect of ethanol, but not that of phenobarbitone in a test of motility in rats.[2] Together these findings clearly show that in a number of paradigms RO 15-4513 is not a selective antagonist of ethanol's actions, but also will reverse those of barbiturates. This is highlighted by a recent report in which RO 15-4513 was found to reverse pentobarbital- but not ethanol-induced hypothermia.[7] It should be noted that RO 15-4513 is a complete and potent benzodiazepine antagonist.[5,6] Whether RO 15-4513 will antagonize the effects of other sedatives acting at other receptors (e.g., histamine receptors) is in need of investigation.

Several of the studies discussed previously provide evidence that RO 15-4513 is not an effective alcohol antagonist in all behavioral paradigms (e.g., it does not appear to oppose hypothermia caused by ethanol[7]). Moreover, in some tests the antagonism of ethanol's effects appears to be virtually complete (e.g., chloride-flux, Vogel conflict test and intoxication ratings[3]) whereas in others the antagonism is only partial (seizure threshold, locomotor stimulation[5,6,8]).

There may also be a species difference in the ability of RO 15-4513 to reverse alcohol's effects. The compound appears to have quite a marked effect on ethanol-induced intoxication in rats,[3] exerts some effect in squirrel-monkeys,[9] but its effects on observer-rated intoxication in mice are less marked (Lister and Nutt, unpublished observations). Although it would be of interest to know whether this compound works in humans, the fact that it is proconvulsant,[9,10] and anxiogenic,[11] and causes seizures in alcohol withdrawal,[12] makes such studies ethically impossible.

Perhaps the most important issue (see Table 1) is whether RO 15-4513's ability to reverse some of ethanol's effects is a result of its action as a partial inverse agonist at central benzodiazepine receptors. Inverse agonists are drugs which bind to the benzodiazepine receptor but which have effects opposite to those of the benzodiazepines (i.e., are proconvulsant and anxiogenic[13]). Certainly RO 15-4513's effects (including alcohol antagonism) appear to be mediated by benzodiazepine receptors, since they are reversed by benzodiazepine antagonists.[2,3,7,11,16] In a number of paradigms, other benzodiazepine receptor inverse agonists at equivalent doses, are capable of reversing some of ethanol's effects.[8,15] There have, however, been reports that some inverse agonists may not be as effective as RO 15-4513 in other paradigms.[2,3] Whether this apparent selectivity is a result of RO 15-4513 acting at some site different from the β-carbolines remains to be determined.

In conclusion, the reversal of some of ethanol's effects by RO 15-4513 has revived interest in ethanol's interactions with the ben-

TABLE 1. Effectiveness of RO 15-4513 compared with other benzodiazepine receptor inverse agonists in antagonising the effects of ethanol [+ = effective, − = ineffective].

test	Ro 15-4513	FG 7142 & other inverse agonists
intoxication (rat)	+	−
horizontal wire	+	−
chloride flux (rat cortex)	+	−
seizure threshold	+	+
exploratory behaviour	+	+
anxiety reduction	+	+
provokes seizures	+	+

zodiazepine/GABA receptor complex. Whether any clinically useful agent will be developed as a result if still a matter of conjecture.[17]

REFERENCES

1. Bonetti EP, Burkard WP, Gabl M, Mohler H. The partial inverse benzodiazepine agonist RO 15-4513 antagonises acute ethanol effects in mice and rats. Br J Pharmacol, 1985; 86:463P.

2. Polc P. Interactions of partial inverse benzodiazepine agonists RO 15-4513 and FG 7142 with ethanol in rats and cats. Br J Pharmacol, 1985; 86:465P.

3. Suzdak P, Glowa JR, Crawley JN, Schwartz RD, Skolnick P, Paul SM. A selective imidazodiazepine antagonist of ethanol in the rat. Science, 1986; 234:1243-1247.

4. Britton KT, Ehlers CL, Koob GF. Ethanol antagonist RO 15-4513 is not selective for ethanol. Science, 1988; 239:648-649.

5. Nutt DJ, Lister RG. The effect of imidazodiazepine RO 15-4513 on the anticonvulsant effects of diazepam, sodium pentobarbital and ethanol. Brain Res, 1987; 413:193-196.

6. Lister RG. Interactions of RO 15-4513 with diazepam, sodium pentobarbital and ethanol in a holeboard test. Pharmacol Biochem Behav, 1987; 28:75-79.

7. Hoffmann PL, Tabakoff B, Szabo G, Suzdak P, Paul SM. Effect of an imidazodiazepine, RO 15-4513, on the incoordination and hypothermia produced by ethanol and pentobarbital. Life Sci, 1987; 41:611-619.

8. Lister RG. The benzodiazepine receptor inverse agonists FG 7142 and RO 15-4513 both reverse some of the behavioral effects of ethanol in a holeboard test. Life Sci, 1987; 41:1481-1489.

9. Miczek KA, Weerts EM. Seizures in drug-treated animals. Science, 1987; 235:1127.

10. Lister RG, Nutt DJ. Interactions of the imidazodiazepine RO 15-4513 with chemical convulsants. Br J Pharmacol, 1988; 93:210-214.

11. Harris CM, Benjamin D, Lal H. Anxiety-like subjective effect of ethanol antagonist RO 15-4513 demonstrated in pentylenetetrazol discrimination. Neuropharmacology, 1987; 26:1545-1547.

12. Lister RG, Karanian J. RO 15-4513 induces seizures in DBA/2 mice undergoing alcohol withdrawal. Alcohol, 1987; 4:409-411.

13. Nutt DJ. Pharmacological and behavioural studies of benzodiazepine antagonists and contragonists. In: Biggio G, Costa E. (eds.) Benzodiazepine recognition site ligands: Biochemistry and Pharmacology. Eds. Adv Biochem Psychopharmacol Raven Press, New York, 1983; 38:153-174.

14. Lister RG. Reversal of the intrinsic effects of RO 15-4513 on exploratory behavior by two benzodiazepine receptor antagonists. Neurosci Letters, in press.

15. Koob GF, Braestrup C, Britton KT. The effects of FG 7142 and RO 15-

1788 on the release of punished responding produced by chlordiazepoxide and ethanol in the rat. Psychopharmacology, 1986; 90:173-178.

16. Sieghart W, Eichinger A, Richards JG, Mohler H. Photoaffinity labeling of benzodiazepine receptor proteins with the partial inverse agonist [3H]Ro 15-4513: a biochemical and autoradiographic study. J Neurochem, 1987; 48:46-52.

17. Lister RG, Nutt DJ. Is RO 15-4513 a specific alcohol antagonist? Trends in Neurosci, 1987; 10:223-225.

GC/MS Assay of Prostaglandins in Cerebrospinal Fluid from Humans and Monkeys

James A. Yergey, PhD
Norman Salem, Jr., PhD
John W. Karanian, PhD
Markku Linnoila, MD, PhD

SUMMARY. The objective of this project has been to develop a sensitive and specific assay for prostaglandins in human cerebrospinal fluid (CSF) from patients with alcoholism and appropriate controls using gas chromatography/mass spectrometry. This study was initiated because numerous literature reports strongly suggest that a relationship exists between ethanol's central nervous system effects and the central production of prostaglandins. In both human and animal studies, administration of prostaglandin synthesis inhibitors prior to administration of ethanol attenuated central nervous system effects of ethanol.

Samples from alcoholics after a three week period of abstinence and normals contained none of the measured prostaglandins (PGE$_2$, PGE$_1$, PGF$_{1a}$, PGF$_{2a}$, 6-keto-PGF$_{1a}$) at a concentration more than twice the limit of quantification (3 pg/mL CSF). Comparison of GC/MS and radioimmunoassay methods provided further validation for these results. Literature reports of much higher levels of prostaglandins in normal controls, i.e., tens to hundreds of pg/mL CSF, appear to be incorrect. Examination of monkey CSF provided a positive control, since several of the prostaglandins were easily quantifiable in these samples.

The authors are affiliated with the Laboratory of Clinical Studies, Division of Intramural Clinical and Biological Research, National Institute on Alcohol Abuse and Alcoholism, NIH Clinical Center, Bldg. 10, Rm. 3C218, Bethesda, MD 20892.

Reprint requests should be sent to James A. Yergey.

INTRODUCTION

A relationship between the central nervous system effects of ethanol and the production of prostaglandins is suggested by the results of several investigators.[1-5] In humans and in animal models, treatment with prostaglandin synthesis inhibitors has been shown to attenuate the central effects of ethanol, including such phenomena as cognitive impairment and withdrawal symptoms. Direct measurements of prostaglandin levels in patients with alcoholism were, therefore, indicated. The principal objective of this study was to develop a sensitive and specific assay for prostaglandins in human cerebrospinal fluid (CSF) collected from patients with alcoholism and appropriate controls, using state-of-the-art gas chromatographic/mass spectrometric (GC/MS) methodologies.

METHODS

Human Cerebrospinal Fluid Assay

The 22-23 mL portion of a 30 mL cerebrospinal fluid sample was drawn into polypropylene tubes. The tubes contained indomethacin to inhibit prostaglandin formation. Exactly 2 mL was transferred to a second tube containing internal standards (250 pg each of tetra-deuterated PGE_2, PGF_{2a}, and 6-keto-PGF_{1a}), and was frozen at $-70°C$. Thawed samples were acidified to pH 3.5 with formic acid and extracted using 1 mL Supelclean LC-18 cartridges as follows: samples were applied, rinsed with 2 mL of 20% methanol, dried for 5 min with nitrogen, rinsed with 2 mL of benzene, and the prostaglandins eluted in 2 mL of methanol directly into silanized glass vials for derivatization. Extracted samples were derivatized to the methoxime, pentafluorobenzyl ester, trimethysilyl ether, and assayed by capillary gas chromatography/negative chemical ionization mass spectrometry using cold on-column injection. The PFB ester thus produced an electronegative species which is favorable for efficient electron capture in a mass spectrometer ion source operated in negative chemical ionization mode, providing further selectivity to the method. The mass spectrometer was operated in selected ion monitoring mode, i.e., only the masses corresponding to the major ion for each prostaglandin were monitored, thus greatly increasing the sensitivity of the technique. Quantification of the prostaglandins was made by comparison to signals for the tetra-deuterated standards added to the sample. Limits of quantification were 3 pg/mL for PGE_2, PGE_1, PGF_{2a}, PGF_{1a}, and 6-keto-PGF_{1a}.

Radioimmunoassay (RIA) – GC/MS Comparison

CSF samples which had been stored without prior addition of tetradeuterated internal standards were extracted and assayed by both methods for PGE_2 and 6-keto-PGF_{1a}. Duplicate CSF samples, collected at the same time, were spiked with 13 pg/mL of both prostaglandins, extracted, and again assayed by both methods.

Monkey CSF Samples

Rhesus monkey CSF samples were collected and were assayed in the same manner as human samples. This nonhuman primate source of CSF offers the possibility of obtaining larger samples volumes and sampling over time.

RESULTS AND DISCUSSION

Patient CSF

Levels of the measured prostaglandins (PGE_2, PGE_1, PGF_{2a}, PGF_{1a}, and 6-keto-PGF_{1a}) in human cerebrospinal fluid from normal controls and alcoholics following 3 weeks abstinence were near or below the limit of quantification. The concentration of 6-keto-PGF_{1a} was measurable in many of the samples, but was never more than twice the limit of quantification. Internal standards were recovered in good yield, ($> 75\%$), indicating that sample storage, extraction, and derivatization were proceeding reliably.

Radioimmunoassay (RIA) – GC/MS Comparison

Unspiked CSF samples contained no quantifiable PGE_2 or 6-keto-PGF_{1a} by either method. Both methods were able to detect the 13 pg/mL increase in prostaglandin level, after the samples were spiked with authentic standards, with acceptable precision and accuracy $[14 \pm 2$ pg/mL (RIA) and 12 ± 3 pg/mL (GC/MS)]. Both methods can, therefore, be used reliably in our laboratory for the measurement of prostaglandins in CSF.

Monkey CSF

Several of the assayed prostaglandins were present in each of the monkey samples at much higher concentrations than in the human CSF, i.e., greater than 100 pg/mL for PGE_2, PGF_{2a}, and 6-keto-PGF_{1a}. These samples provided a positive control, indicating that endogenously produced prostaglandins were indeed quantifiable using our methodologies.

CONCLUSIONS

The levels of the five prostaglandins measured in human cerebrospinal fluid from normal individuals and alcoholics following three weeks of abstinence are near or below the 3 pg/mL level. Literature reports of much higher levels in normal controls, i.e., tens to hundreds of pg/mL appear to be incorrect. A positive control for the measurement of endogenously produced prostaglandins was found upon examining several CSF samples from rhesus monkeys. Studies on circadian production of prostaglandins are in progress. It is hoped that these studies might help to explain the very low levels measured thus far in the human samples. Studies in progress will quantify the prostaglandin levels in CSF in drinking alcoholics and alcoholics during acute withdrawal.

REFERENCES

1. Linnoila M, Seppala T, Mattila MJ. Acute effect of antipyretic analgesics, alone or in combination with alcohol, on human psychomotor skills related to driving. Br J Clin Pharmac. 1974; 1:477-484.

2. Collier HOJ, Hammond MD, Schneider C. Effects of drugs affecting endogenous amines or cyclic nucleotides on ethanol withdrawal head twitches in mice. Br J Pharmac. 1976; 58:9-16.

3. George FR, Collins AC. Ethanol's behavioral effects may be partly due to increases in brain prostaglandin production. Alc Clin Exp Res. 1985; 9:143-146.

4. Grupp LA, Elias J, Perlanski E, Stewart RB. Modification of ethanol-induced motor impairment by diet, diuretic, mineralocorticoid, or prostaglandin synthetase inhibitor, Psychopharm. 1985; 87:20-24.

5. Minocha A, Barth JT, Herold DA, Gideon DA, Spyker DA. Modulation of ethanol induced central nervous system depression by ibuprofen. Clin Pharmacol Ther. 1986; 39:123-127.

Ethanol, Its Metabolism
and Gonadal Effects:
Does Sex Make a Difference?

David H. Van Thiel, MD
Ralph E. Tarter, PhD
Elaine Rosenblum, MS
Judith S. Gavaler, PhD

SUMMARY. The role of gender as a variable that might affect the metabolism of ethanol and thus the consequences of ethanol metabolism is reviewed. First, the pharmacodynamics of ethanol are reviewed. Specific differences between males and females relative to ethanol pharmacokinetic parameters are discussed including gender differences in the volume of distribution and putative hormonal effects on achieved blood alcohol levels. In addition, attention is directed toward the metabolic capacity of alcohol dehydrogenase and

---

David H. Van Thiel is with the Division of Gastroenterology, Department of Medicine and Ralph E. Tarter is with the Department of Psychiatry, the University of Pittsburgh, School of Medicine, Pittsburgh, PA 15261. Elaine Rosenblum and Judith S. Gavaler are also affiliated with the University of Pittsburgh, School of Medicine.

Reprint requests should be directed to David H. Van Thiel.

This work supported in part by NIAAA AA06601, NIDDKD AM32556, NIAAA AA06772, NIAAA AA04425.

131

the microsomal ethanol oxidizing system with respect to effects of both sex differences and hormonal manipulations on the activities of these ethanol metabolizing enzymes. Finally, the data upon which the concept of sex-related differences in susceptibility to alcohol induced end organ failure are presented.

PHARMACOLOGY OF ETHANOL

Absorption

Ethanol is a small, moderately polar, readily diffusible molecule that is infinitely soluble in water. Once ingested, it enters the body from the stomach and intestine by simple diffusion.[1,2] Once absorbed, it distributes in total body water and is oxidized within the liver to carbon dioxide and water. Only minor amounts are excreted unmetabolized in urine, breath and sweat. No known feedback regulation of ethanol metabolism exists. Thus, for any given amount ingested, its metabolism continues until there is no longer any ethanol left.[2]

Ethanol absorption is greater from the intestine than from the stomach. This reflects the anatomic and physiologic differences that exist between these two gastrointestinal organs. In general, the stomach acts as a reservoir and mixer of ingested food and beverage. It predigests protein and grinds solids to a near liquid state (chyme) and then releases the chyme to the small bowel as an isotonic semi-liquid mixture with a rather uniform caloric density. In general, alcoholic beverages are hyperosmolar. Under normal conditions they delay gastric emptying until the osmolarity of the gastric content approaches isotonicity. Once emptied into the small intestine, the absorption of ethanol is rapid. The absorption of the nonethanolic components of the material released by the stomach to the small bowel lags behind that of ethanol as a function of the time required for their complete digestion by pancreatic and intestinal enzymes. Once totally digested, they also are absorbed either passively or via carriers that are specific for individual classes of amino acids, small peptides, sugars or fatty acids.

Additional factors that affect gastric emptying and alter the rate of intestinal or pancreatic digestion of intestinal content can alter the pharmacokinetics of ethanol absorption and metabolism. Specifically, prior gastric surgery can either enhance or, more usually, delay gastric emptying. Such surgery also allows hyperosmolar material such as alcoholic beverages to enter the intestine prior to its conversion to an isotonic fluid mixture. As a result, intestinal absorption of ethanol is hastened due to a greater luminal concentration (the driving force for passive absorption) as well as the production of a leakier intestinal membrane as a result of ethanol and hyperosmolar-induced intestinal injury.

Women have been shown to have different rates of gastric emptying and oral-cecal intestinal transit times as a function of the menstrual cycle and pregnancy.[3-9] Specifically, the luteal phase of the menstrual cycle, which is characterized by high estradiol and progesterone levels, and pregnancy, which is also characterized by high estradiol and progesterone levels, have been shown to be associated with reduced gastrointestinal motility and prolonged gastrointestinal transit times. As a result, gastric emptying and intestinal transit are delayed in women during the luteal phase, or pregnancy, as compared with the follicular phase of the menstrual cycle. Moreover, the increased progesterone levels characteristic of the luteal phase of the menstrual cycle and pregnancy have been shown to be the agent responsible for these alterations both *in vivo* as well as *in vitro* studies.[5-9] No such cyclic changes occur in males. As a result, ethanol delivery to the intestine and subsequently to the vascular system is not as variable in men as it is in women.

Ethanol Pharmacodynamics

Ethanol is usually taken orally. Thus, before it enters the systemic circulation it undergoes some fractional metabolism by the intestinal tract, its bacterial and fungal populations, and the liver. This first pass effect can be significant. In individuals who abuse ethanol, this first pass effect may be greater than that experienced by ethanol-naive individuals as a result of enzyme induction, particularly induction of the mixed function oxidase activity of the intestine and liver. The first pass effect in individuals with portal hypertension may be greatly reduced as a result of the shunting of portal venous ethanol-enriched blood away from the liver and into the systemic circulation.

The most basic relationship in pharmacokinetics is that between the dose of a drug and the blood level that results after its administration; the volume of distribution of a drug (V_d) is the volume in which a given dose must be distributed in order to obtain the level of the drug observed immediately after its intravenous administration. Thus, the V_d is equal to the dose divided by the attained plasma concentration. Typically, compared to men, women have smaller volumes of distribution for water soluble drugs like ethanol and larger volumes of distribution for fat soluble drugs. Once absorbed, most drugs, including ethanol, are eliminated from the plasma in direct proportion to their plasma concentrations (i.e., they obey first-order kinetics). Therefore, the plasma concentration-time curve provides a simple way to calculate the effectiveness of oral drug administration. The area under the plasma concentration-time curve is directly related to the dose given; the ratio of the area under the curve (AUC) achieved by oral administration to the area produced by an identical intravenous dose yields the bioavailability of the drug. The difference between these two areas yields the amount metabolized as a result of the first pass effect.

Ethanol Metabolism

Once absorbed and presented to the liver, ethanol metabolism begins; two major enzyme systems are responsible for the hepatic metabolism of ethanol.[1,2] These are the cytosolic enzyme, alcohol dehydrogenase (ADH), which is responsible for 80-85% of the metabolism of ethanol, and the microsomal mixed function oxidase or microsomal ethanol oxidizing system (MEOS) which is responsible for 10-15% of the metabolism of ethanol. The first of these two enzymes has a low Km for ethanol of approximately 1.0 mM and is active at all concentrations seen under physiologic conditions.[2] In contrast, the MEOS system has a Km for ethanol in the 10 mM or greater range and is active when higher levels of ethanol exist in the blood.[10-13] Importantly, being a cytosolic enzyme, ADH is not inducible. In contrast, MEOS, being a microsomal enzyme, is inducible and is found in greater amounts in the liver of chronic alcoholics and alcohol-fed animals as well as in those who use cross-tolerant drugs.[10-13]

SPECIFIC DIFFERENCES BETWEEN MALES AND FEMALES

Sex Differences in Various Ethanol Pharmacokinetic Parameters

Rats decrease their voluntary ethanol intake while receiving estrogens parenterally.[14,15] They also ingest less ethanol during estrus than at other times in the menstrual cycle.[15,16]

In contrast, the administration of exogenous androgens and progesterone does not alter the voluntary intake of ethanol by rats.[17,18]

Similarly in humans, Little et al., have shown that there is a sharp decrease in alcoholic beverage consumption during pregnancy, and that this voluntary reduction in ethanol intake occurs both in alcoholic as well as in nonalcoholic women.[19,20]

A similar observation has been made by Zeiner and Kegg who noted in American Indian women, matched for age, education, socioeconomic level and body habitus, that the use of oral contraceptives (pseudopregnancy) was associated with a significantly reduced voluntary intake of ethanol as compared to that found in women not ingesting such drugs.[21,23]

Jones and Jones have compared the pharmacokinetics of ethanol administration in men and women as well as in women during different phases of the menstrual cycle.[24-27] They found that women, as compared to men, exhibited higher peak blood alcohol concentrations (BAC) and that the greatest BACs were achieved in women studied just prior to menstruation.

Zeiner et al. extended these studies and examined the effect of oral contraceptive use (pseudopregnancy) on ethanol pharmacokinetics and acetaldehyde levels in Caucasian women and compared the responses observed with those obtained in normal female controls not ingesting oral contraceptives.[21-23] As in the studies of Jones and Jones, they administered 0.52 grams of ethanol per kg of body weight to each of their subjects at two points in the drug controlled menstrual cycle. In contrast to the observations reported by Jones and Jones, however, they found a greater peak BAC when estrogen and progesterone levels were low rather than when both estrogen and progesterone levels were high. Interestingly, blood acetaldehyde levels were greater when BACs were lower and when estrogen and progesterone levels were greater than when both hormone levels were at low levels.

Marshall et al. performed the most comprehensive study of the pharmacokinetics of ethanol metabolism in women (both during the follicular and luteal phases of the menstrual cycle) and in men.[28] They demonstrated clearly that the ethanol concentration-time profiles in women during both halves of the menstrual cycle are similar, and that no difference in mean total body water is discernible between the follicular and luteal phases of the menstrual cycle. In contrast, the mean ethanol concentration-time curves in males and females differ significantly, although the time required to reach peak BACs does not differ between the sexes. The mean peak ethanol concentrations and the mean area under the curve (AUC) of the ethanol concentration-time plot were significantly greater in females than they were in males. This difference was due entirely to the difference between the volumes of distribution (V_dd) of ethanol in men and women. In males, mean body water expressed as a percentage of body weight ($65 \pm 2\%$) was significantly greater than it was in females ($51 \pm 2\%$). Moreover, as might be expected, a significant correlation was found between the volumes of distribution of ethanol and of total body water. They also found a significant inverse relationship between the ethanol concentration-time AUC and total body water for both males and females. Several other investigators have confirmed various individual components of the more extensive studies of Marshall et al.[28-33] Taken together, these data strongly suggest that sex differences in total body water, ethanol V_d, and the ethanol concentration-time AUC can be accounted for by of the difference between the body water contents of the two sexes. These data also help to explain why women appear to develop greater degrees of hepatic injury than do males when their ethanol intake has been adjusted for body weight; in such circumstances, the peak blood alcohol concentration achieved in women would be greater than those achieved in males.

The effect of the menstrual cycle and hormone status on the psychological effects of alcohol use are extremely controversial.[26,34-39] Jones and Jones did not find neuropsychological performance differences as a function of the menstrual cycle in women ingesting alcohol.[35] In contrast, Linnoila et al. found no effect of blood alcohol concentration as a function of the menstrual cycle, but they did find a positive correlation between blood alcohol concentrations and reaction time impairments;[36] interestingly, this association was seen only during the luteal phase of the menstrual cycle when estrogen and progesterone levels are both high. Sutker et al., studied 32 adult women over a period of time encompassed by two complete menstrual cycles and estimated the degree of anxiety, depression, and hostility experienced by the individuals studied.[40] They found that each of these mood states correlated highly with the others but that negative moods did not appear to relate to either the frequency or amount of alcohol ingested. They did determine, however, that normally cycling women reported more frequent drinking to relieve tension/depression during menses than at other times in the menstrual cycle.

Sex Differences in Ethanol Metabolism

Rachamin et al. were the first to examine the effects of sex hormone alterations and pubertal development on the hepatic activity of alcohol dehydrogenase (ADH) and the rate of ethanol metabolism in male and female animals.[41] They found that prepubertal animals of both sexes had high hepatic ADH activity (250-350 mg of ethanol/hr/kg), whereas adult animals of both sexes had considerably lower levels of activity. Specifically, they found that adult female animals had greater hepatic ADH activity (210-335 mg ethanol/hr/kg) than did adult male animals (110-130 mg ethanol/hr/kg) ($p < 0.01$). Moreover, they noted that, as the hepatic activity of ADH fell in male rats as they matured, so did their ability to catabolize ethanol. Castration of male rats prevented the decrease in ethanol clearance and hepatic ADH activity in normal male rats whereas ovariectomy had no effect upon female rats.

The chronic administration of testosterone to castrated male rats as well as to female rats reduced their rates of ethanol metabolism to levels found in mature males.[41] In contrast, the administration of estradiol to male rats produced a marked enhancement of ethanol metabolism and hepatic ADH activity in mature adult male animals. Moreover, the administration of ethanol to prepubertal male rats (presumably by preventing puberty) prevented the fall in ethanol metabolic rates and hepatic ADH activity noted in normal male rats as they progress through puberty.

Mezey and associates have extended the *in vivo* studies of Rachamin with *in vitro* studies using isolated hepatocytes maintained in tissue culture.[42-44] They showed that dihydrotestosterone (DHT), but not testosterone, is responsible for the suppression of ADH activity and the ethanol elimination capacity observed in hepatocytes obtained from adult male rats.[43]

These authors noted that DHT, at high unphysiological levels, is both a substrate for ADH in the reductive direction and an inhibitor of ethanol oxidation by ADH.[42] The Ki of DHT for the inhibition of ethanol oxidation, however is 11.5 uM, which is ten times greater than the physiologic concentration of the hormone in blood. A more likely mechanism for the observed effect of DHT in suppressing hepatic ADH activity may be an effect of the steroid upon enzyme degradation. Mezey has been able to demonstrate that an enhancement in the rate of ADH degradation occurs in males, when compared to females; that it is due to the presence of DHT in the male; and that the fall in levels of DHT which occur with castration is the principal cause for the increase in ADH activity seen in adult male rat liver following castration.

These studies are important because they contribute substantially to our understanding of the mechanisms that regulate alcohol dehydrogenase activity and therefore ethanol metabolism. These factors include the nutritional state of the individual, the level of ADH activity in the liver, and the rate of reoxidation of NADH within the liver cell.

The parallel changes in the dehydrogenase activity reported by Mezey et al.[41-44] suggest that ADH is the major determinant of the rate of ethanol oxidation present under normal circumstances within the liver. This conclusion is substantiated further by the parallel decrease in ethanol elimination observed in association with inhibition of ADH activity seen with 4-methylpyrazole administration. Moreover, the failure to observe a significant change in ethanol elimination with the addition of substrates for the malate-aspartate shuttle or in the presence of an uncoupler of oxidative phosphorylation suggest that mitochondrial transfer of or oxidation of NADH is not rate limiting for ethanol oxidation.[42-44]

Mezey and associates have examined the effects of ovariectomy and estrogen administration on the hepatic level of ADH activity in female rats. Estradiol administration increased hepatic weight and total ADH activity per liver but not per gram liver. In contrast, ovariectomy had no effect on hepatic ADH activity or on ethanol elimination capacity. These data suggest that, under the circumstances of the experimental models used, factors other than total enzyme activity, such as the rate of reoxidation of NADH, are rate limiting for ethanol oxidation. The specific reasons for the differences observed in this regard with adult male and female hepatocytes, studied either *in vivo* or *in vitro*, remain to be specifically determined.

Sex steroids have variable effects on microsomal drug metabolizing systems.[45-48] In general, females have an increased net reductive activity whereas males have an increased net oxidative activity of their hepatic mixed function oxidase activity.[49] Moreover, pregnancy has been shown to be associated with a reduced ability to metabolize drugs. Estrogen administration and the use of oral contraceptive agents have been shown to diminish hepatic drug metabolism of a wide variety of model drugs.[48-53]

The hepatic activity of the microsomal ethanol oxidizing system (MEOS) has been shown to be sex hormone dependent by Teschke and Heymann. These investigators have shown that castration of adult male rats leads to a striking reduction of the hepatic activity of MEOS. The administration of exogenous testosterone to castrate males completely restores MEOS activity to that present in intact males. As with castration, estradiol administration results in diminished hepatic MEOS activity.[13,54,55]

Castration of male rats also reduces the hepatic content of microsomal cytochrome P-450 and NADPH cytochrome c reductase. As was the case with MEOS, the reduction in microsomal cytochrome P-450 and NADPH cytochrome c reductase associated with castration can be prevented by the administration of exogenous testosterone.[54]

In contrast, although hepatic microsomal cytochrome P-450 in the liver of adult male animals can be reduced, no change in microsomal cytochrome c reductase activity is produced by estradiol administration. This latter finding suggests that the activity of microsomal cytochrome c reductase activity is not rate limiting for MEOS activity. These findings, particularly in terms of the effect that MEOS activity has upon both acetaldehyde production within the cell and lipid peroxidation, raise important questions as to the extent that these alterations in alcohol dehydrogenase and MEOS activity may play in the well established enhanced susceptibility of females to alcohol associated hepatic injury.

SEX DIFFERENCES IN ETHANOL INGESTION RATES AND ETHANOL-INDUCED LIVER DISEASE

In a classical international temporal trend analysis, Joliffe and Jellinek demonstrated a significant association between changes in the consumption of alcoholic beverages and changes in cirrhosis rates.[56] Although challenged initially, later studies have strengthened the association between national alcohol use rates and cirrhosis rates.[56-60] Thus, most recent studies have chosen not to examine the association between liver disease and alcohol ingestion rates in the population generally but instead have examined the differences between men and women for these two factors and the relationships between them.

Presently, there are more than 10 reports from many different groups, which suggest that sex-related differences in alcohol-induced liver disease exist.[61-71] Each of these studies used different methodological designs, was performed at different points of time, examined quite different patient populations, and involved subjects in at least five different countries. The consistency of the findings strongly suggest that actual differences in alcohol associated hepatic disease risk exist between the two sexes.

Spain was one of the first authors to note a difference in susceptibility to alcohol-induced hepatic disease of women, compared to men.[70] He examined the necropsy records of patients who underwent autopsy over a seven year period between 1936 and 1942 at Bellevue Hospital in New York City. He found 250 cases of cirrhosis among the 5495 post-mortem exams performed during this period. One-hundred and ninety of the cirrhotics were male and 60 were female. The 3:1 sex ratio of cirrhosis reflected the male to female ratio among those necropsied for all causes of death at the hospital during the same period. Interestingly, the mean age at the time of death due to alcoholic liver disease was eight years younger for the females than it was for the males studied. More impressive was the finding that the mean age for those who died of cirrhosis or its complications was 10.5 years older for males than it was for the females studied. Equally impressive, if not more so, was the finding that there was a predominance of males among those who died with cirrhosis or succumbed to complications related to the presence of portal hypertension, whereas the females more frequently died as a direct result of hepatocellular failure. In an attempt to eliminate the possibility of an age factor as the underlying cause for this difference, he then examined only males less than 50 years of age at death and compared the causes of death in this group of males to those in the cirrhotic women, all of whom were less than 50 years of age at the time of their death. With this correction, the percentage of males who died of causes unrelated to hepatic failure or to its complications rose to a level three times that seen in the females studied.

Twenty-four years later, Wilkinson et al. reported their findings on 800 chronic alcoholics attending an alcoholism clinic in Melbourne, Australia.[61] Twice as many women as men had cirrhosis when first seen at the clinic ($p < 0.05$). More importantly, when the cirrhotic men and women were compared, the women were found to have started drinking eight years later than had the men ($p < 0.01$); the women drank excessively for a shorter period of time (nine years) than had the men (21 years) ($p < 0.01$). Further, the women drank an average of 70 grams of ethanol less per day while drinking excessively, yet still had a two fold greater rate of cirrhosis while being nearly identical in age at time of presentation to the clinic when compared to males.

In a second paper by the same group evaluating 1000 alcoholics seen in Australia the finding of cirrhosis was twice as common in women as it was in men. This despite the fact that the women presented at the same age as did the men while having begun to drink at a later age and having drank 95g of ethanol/day less on average than did the men studied, and having admitted to ethanol abuse for less time (12 years) as compared to the males (18 years) (all statistically significant).[62]

Confirming the above findings Peguignot et al., while attempting to examine the risk of cirrhosis as a function of increasing doses of ethanol in French subjects, reported important differences in the alcohol-dose response curves for males and females.[71] In their study, the findings on 227 hospitalized alcoholic cirrhotics and 2000 nonhospitalized controls between the ages of 45 and 74 were compared. Among the males studied, the mean daily alcohol consumption was 132g/day in the cirrhotics and 50g/day in the controls. Particularly important to note is the finding that the daily intake of ethanol among hospitalized alcoholic cirrhotic women was essentially identical to that of the nonhospitalized control male population. The authors then calculated a morbidity index for each dose of ethanol. At levels of ingestion less than 60g in men and 20g in women, the risk of cirrhosis was minimal. At levels above these cut off points, the risk of cirrhosis increased rapidly for both sexes but was three times as rapid in females as it was in males. It is particularly important to note that the cut off point in males for no risk for cirrhosis was 10g/day above the mean daily intake found in hospitalized *cirrhotic* women.

Morgan and Sherlock have reported their observations relative to sex related differences in 100 consecutive patients with alcohol related liver disease observed in a single year at their institution.[69] They found that women were less likely to be suspected of alcohol abuse, even when they developed withdrawal symptoms in the hospital. Moreover, they noted that women presented with more advanced histologic disease despite a similar length of alcohol use and age at presentation as compared to the men seen. Specifically, female alcoholics were more likely ($p < 0.05$) to present in hepatic failure, to have evidence of peripheral neuropathy ($p < 0.025$), cerebellar ataxia ($p < 0.05$) and alcoholic psychosis ($p < 0.05$) than the alcoholic men seen at their institution. These findings suggest, but do not prove, that women are more susceptible to alcohol-related hepatic disease than are men when ethanol intakes are similar. The previously described studies have been most carefully reviewed and critically analyzed in a particularly thoughtful review published in 1982.[63]

The factors influencing the histological evolution of alcoholic hepatitis without cirrhosis were evaluated in 14 males and 12 female patients who were followed for a minimum of five years in Spain.[66] Half of the total group discontinued their intake of alcohol during the study period, while four others reduced their daily intake of ethanol markedly. At the end of the study period, no significant differences in age, sex, amount of alcohol intake, clinical data, results of liver function tests and histological severity of alcoholic hepatitis at the time of initial diagnosis were noted between patients abstaining or not abstaining. There were however marked differences in the histological outcome of liver lesions between the various groups. Four of the 13 who stopped drinking progressed to cirrhosis while the last liver biopsy in the remaining nine showed histologic improvement. Improvement in the liver lesion was noted in all of the four patients who reduced their alcohol intake. In contrast, the nine patients who continued to drink large amounts of ethanol progressed to cirrhosis while four still had alcoholic hepatitis. Seven of the 12 women, but only two of the 14 men, progressed to cirrhosis ($p < 0.02$). Importantly, the progression to cirrhosis in women was not found to be related to the continued use of ethanol. These data suggest that once a certain level of alcohol induced hepatic injury occurs in women it continues independently of whether or not the women continue to ingest alcohol. Such an observation would have important clinical implications should it be confirmed in future studies.

RECOGNITION OF ALCOHOL EFFECTS ON ENDOCRINE FUNCTION

Background

That alcoholic beverage use and abuse can produce reproductive dysfunction has long been recognized. Well before even the vaguest recognition of either the role of gametes or the concept of hormones, abuse of alcoholic beverages was noted to have an adverse effect on reproductive capability.

Not surprisingly, the endocrine effects of chronic alcoholic beverage abuse were first reported in alcoholic males with Laennec's (alcohol-induced) cirrhosis. Essentially all of these early reports were based on observational studies in males, and later experimental studies were also performed exclusively in males. This early reliance on study populations composed only of males reflects two realities: Males, but not females, were readily available for both observational and experimental studies; the external aspects of male, but not of female, reproductive function are such that the endocrine sequelae of alcoholic beverage abuse were easily detectable in males.

There was little disagreement among early investigators that alcoholic cirrhotic males manifested signs of endocrine dysfunction. During the last half of the 19th century and the first half of this century, however, the malnutrition associated with alcoholism was presumed to be the cause of the observed cirrhosis. Further, the presence of cirrhosis, rather than alcoholic beverage abuse per se was considered to be the major factor responsible for both the hypogonadism and feminization.

DUALITY OF ALCOHOL EFFECTS: HYPOGONADISM AND FEMINIZATION

Little progress was made in elucidating the effects of alcoholic beverage abuse on endocrine function until the syndromes of hypogonadism and feminization were conceptually separated. In the male, hypogonadism includes both hypoandrogenization and reproductive failure, whereas the physical findings of feminization include gynecomastia, a female escutcheon, palmar erythema and spider angiomata. Because the early observational studies evaluated alcoholic cirrhotic males in whom the signs of both feminization and hypogonadism were present, it is not surprising that these two syndromes were considered to be a single entity.

With the conceptual dissociation of hypogonadism and feminization, hypotheses were more clearly formulated, and study protocols were designed to evaluate specific components of testable hypotheses. The development of animal models and the use of ethanol as the experimental approximation of alcoholic beverages provided powerful experimental tools. The use of animal models provided a framework within which both the reproductive failure and the endocrine disruption and dysfunction associated with alcoholic beverage abuse could be studied.

In males, the effects of alcohol on the hypothalamic pituitary-gonadal axis have been extensively examined and a variety of intermeshing components of the mechanisms involved have been described. In females, there has been far less progress. This difference in the extent to which alcohol endocrine interactions have yielded to understanding reflects the difference between the sexes in the complexity of gonadal function and regulation of the hypothalamic pituitary gonadal axis.

HYPOGONADISM: DISRUPTION OF GONADAL FUNCTION BY ALCOHOL

The Normal Hypothalamic Pituitary Gonadal Axis

Although the overall function of the gonads is to produce gametes for reproductive purposes and to synthesize sex steroids for the development and maintenance of secondary sex characteristics, the mechanisms by which these functional goals are achieved in each sex are quite different. The gonads of both males and females contain two distinct functional compartments. The reproductive compartment of the male is composed of the seminiferous tubules with their contained developing and mature sperm; this process of active germ cell production occupies up to 95% of the volume of the testes. Millions of mature germ cells (spermatazoa) are produced daily and this daily production usually continues until late adult life and may be unabated until death. The endocrine compartment of the testes is composed of Leydig cells which synthesize and secrete androgens. The Leydig cells occupy less than 5% of total testicular volume. At the hypothalamic pituitary level, the male is characterized neuroendocrinologically by regular bursts of gonadotropin releasing hormone (GnRH) release and rather stable plasma levels of both luteinizing hormone (LH) and follicle stimulating hormone (FSH).

In contrast to the large volume of the male gonad committed to germ cell production, less than 10% of the ovarian volume of adult females during the reproductive years consists of germ cells available for gamete production. Further, unlike the male, the absolute number of germ cells per ovary is fixed even before birth and that number diminishes steadily thereafter as a result of either ovulation or atresia. The endocrine compartment of the ovary occupies a considerable volume of the adult ovary; it consists of three component cell types, each of which is functional as part of the various structures produced during and after the development of a mature ovum. Each of the components of the ovarian endocrine compartment functions at a different rate during the menstrual cycle, and as much as 90% of the biologically active estradiol secreted by the ovary during any given cycle originates from the unique primordial follicle containing the primary oocyte destined for ovulation during that cycle. As the primordial follicle becomes the primary follicle, the granulosa cells of this developing structure synthesize the estrogen which is required for both follicular maturation and the maintenance of female sexual characteristics. As the primary follicle matures to become a Graafian follicle, the contained thecal cells, which produce the androgen precursors of estrogen, augment estrogen production to provide for the burst of gonadotropin secretion essential for ovulation. Following ovulation, the ruptured follicle develops into the component of the endocrine compartment responsible for the production of progesterone, the corpus luteum.

In contrast to the male, the female is characterized by a complex neuroendocrine clock such that gonadotropins are not secreted synchronously and plasma levels vary dramatically in a regular manner which is characteristic of the menstrual cycle. During the normal cycle, plasma LH levels show a slight rise in the late follicular phase, followed by a marked preovulatory surge and then a decline during the luteal phase. The target sites for LH are theca, stromal, and luteal cells, as well as granulosa cells; the target for FSH is exclusively the granulosa cell. Plasma FSH rises during the late luteal and early follicular phases followed by a decline which is interrupted at mid cycle by a small surge coinciding with the preovulatory LH peak.

PERTUBATION OF GONADAL FUNCTION AND HYPOTHALAMIC PITUITARY REGULATION BY ALCOHOL

The Male

Failure of the male reproductive compartment is commonly manifested as testicular atrophy and hypo- or azoospermia. Testicular endocrine failure is manifested by the loss of secondary sex characteristics; in response to reduced testosterone levels, such men become less muscular, lose sexual hair on the face, axilla and pubic areas, have reduced size of prostate, seminal vesicles and phallus, manifest decrements in scrotal wrinkling, and complain of impotence and loss of libido.

Indeed, such were the findings reported in the earliest studies describing the endocrine abnormalities observed in cirrhotic alcoholic males.[72] With the advent of steroid hormone assays, it became clear that the testicular atrophy, impotence and loss of libido in alcoholic males with alcohol-induced liver disease occurred in the presence of decreased circulating testosterone levels;[73-82] it is also to be noted that many of these studies also concomitantly reported findings of feminization in these cirrhotic alcoholics. With the application of animal models and the use of ethanol as the experimental approximation of alcoholic beverages, the fact that testicular failure could be produced in the absence of advanced biochemical and/or histologic liver disease emerged. Specifically, administration of ethanol to mice and rats resulted in reduced numbers of progeny, testicular atrophy, and decrements in plasma testosterone levels, occurring with hepatic histology no more severe than steatosis.[83-93]

With the separation of the concepts of hypogonadism and feminization, followed by the subsequent conceptual dissociation of hypogonadism and putatively obligate liver disease, hypogonadism emerged as an individual entity to be elucidated with respect to alcohol rather than liver disease as the operative variable. Important information was provided via the application of three different clinical approaches. First, studies comparing alcoholic cirrhotic males to males with cirrhosis of a nonalcohol etiology demonstrated that the testicular atrophy and reductions in testosterone were indeed a function of alcohol rather than of cirrhosis per se.[94]

Second, clinical studies in which ethanol was administered to normal male volunteer subjects reported that ethanol administered acutely resulted in a fall in testosterone which occurred synchronously with an appropriate rise in LH, whereas chronic ethanol administration for 4 weeks to normal males resulted in a continued progressive decline of testosterone accompanied by a decrease (rather than an appropriate increase) in LH levels.[95-97] The third clinical approach evaluated abstaining alcoholic males and demonstrated reduced levels of testosterone, but "normal" to moderately increased LH concentrations.[98] Taken together, these clinical data suggested that alcohol ingestion is followed by an initial Leydig cell injury resulting in a reduction in plasma testosterone and an appropriate compensatory increase in gonadotropin levels; with continued alcohol abuse, testosterone levels continue to fall while gonadotropin concentrations return towards paradoxically "normal" levels.

With the link between alcohol and decrements in gonadal endocrine function demonstrated in clinical studies, the animal models could then be exploited to evaluate hypotheses as to the mechanisms involved. Studies using an isolated perfused rat testes preparation demonstrated that ethanol is a direct testicular toxin producing dose-dependent decreases in testicular testosterone production and synthesis.[99] Studies using Leydig cells obtained from both rats and humans, maintained in tissue culture and exposed to stimulatory levels of gonadotropin, demonstrated that testosterone secretion is markedly reduced by the addition of either ethanol or its first metabolic product, acetaldehyde.[100,101] Ethanol, at levels as low as 25 mg/dl (5.4 mM), inhibits rat Leydig cell synthesis and secretion of testosterone by as much as 44%. In passing, it is worth noting that the legal limit defining intoxication is 100 mg/dl. Acetaldehyde is an even more toxic substance and significantly inhibits rat Leydig cell synthesis and secretion of testosterone when added to the culture medium at concentrations as low as 5uM. These studies have provided clear evidence of the toxic effect of both ethanol and of its first metabolic product, acetaldehyde, on the male gonadal endocrine compartment.

Even with the above studies, however, the question of the hypothalamic pituitary failure of gonadotropin release observed in chronic alcoholic men with advanced testicular failure remained. Studies using an inhibitor of ethanol metabolism to maintain sustained high blood alcohol levels have provided additional information.[102] In male rats given the standard alcohol diet to which was added 4-methylpyrazole, an inhibitor of alcohol dehydrogenase, plasma gonadotropin levels do not rise to counteract the decrease in testosterone but rather fall to levels below the normal range; these data suggest that, in this particular model at least, both Leydig cell injury and central hypothalamic pituitary failure of gonadotropin secretion can occur with alcohol abuse if sustained high levels of blood alcohol are maintained.

Morphologic studies have contributed to our knowledge concerning the intracellular mechanisms of alcohol-induced testicular injury. Morphologically, the testes of chronic alcoholic men and of chronic alcohol-fed male rats appear quite similar. Both show advanced germ cell injury with few if any normal residual germ cells within the seminiferous tubules, which are markedly decreased in diameter and are surrounded by a peritubular fibrotic process.[91,93,102-104] At the light microscopic level, the Leydig cells appear to be normal and possibly increased in number. This apparent Leydig cell hyperplasia probably represents the collapse of normal numbers of Leydig cells into groups around residual seminiferous tubules occurring as a consequence of the loss of seminiferous tubular volume. At the electron microscopic level, the Leydig cells of rats chronically fed alcohol appear to be reduced in size, to have a reduced cytoplasmic volume and to demonstrate a relative hypertrophy of the mitochondria, such that individual mitochondria are larger and the fractional volume of the cytopolasmic mass committed to mitochondrial function is increased significantly.[105]

Probably even more important for testosterone biosynthesis, however, is the reduction in the volume of the Leydig cell committed to microsomal function. Moreover, even when one corrects for the reduction in microsomal protein seen in the Leydig cells obtained from rats fed alcohol, ethanol feeding can be shown to reduce the activity of 3-beta-hydroxysteroid dehydrogenase/delta 5-4 isomerase, desmolase, and 17 alpha oxidoreductase, the three microsomal enzymes which are important in steroidogenesis.[86-89,106-110] Not only is the activity of 3-beta-hydroxysteroid dehydrogenase and delta 5-4 isomerase reduced as a consequence of alcohol abuse when tested under ideal conditions of excess cofactors and substrates, but ethanol feeding also alters the testicular redox state in a direction disadvantageous to the activity of this enzyme. More importantly, increases in NADH per se, even in the presence of equimolar increases in NAD, such that the net ratio of NAD to NADH is not disturbed, also inhibits this enzyme complex.[111]

Relevant to this latter issue of increases in NADH and altered redox states occurring as a consequence of alcohol abuse, as well as the effects of acetaldehyde upon Leydig cells, is the relatively recent observation that the testes contain an alcohol dehydrogenase distinct from hepatic alcohol dehydrogenase.[112-115]

Much, although not all, of the activity of the testicular alcohol dehydrogenase is contained within the Leydig cells. The demonstration of this enzyme within the testes provides a mechanism whereby the metabolism of alcohol locally within the testes could thereby alter the testicular redox state by generating locally increased concentrations of the even more toxic product acetaldehyde. Indeed, recent studies demonstrate that chronic ethanol administration to male rats results in measurable changes in testicular mitochondrial diene conjugates, polyenoic fatty acid composition, malonaldehyde formation, and reduced glutathione levels; these findings suggest that lipid peroxidation may also contribute to the testicular injury observed.[116]

Finally, the presence of a testicular alcohol dehydrogenase provides an additional mechanism by which germ cell injury can occur as a consequence of alcohol abuse. Specifically, retinol is essential for normal spermatogenesis. It reaches the testes via the circulation as the retinyl ester and is converted to the free alcohol and then to the aldehyde, retinal, which is the form of the vitamin essential for normal spermatogenesis. Testicular alcohol dehydrogenase not only oxidizes ethanol to acetaldehyde but also converts retinol to retinal.[113,115,117] Moreover, ethanol inhibits the generation of retinal from retinol in a noncompetitive manner. Thus alcohol metabolism by testicular alcohol dehydrogenase contributes importantly to both the

Leydig cell and the germ cell injury associated with alcohol abuse in the male.

THE FEMALE DURING THE REPRODUCTIVE YEARS

If one were to guess that the adverse effects of alcoholic beverage abuse in females during the reproductive years might ultimately result in ovarian failure, then one might expect to see disruption of cyclic ovarian function as manifested by oligomenorrhea, hypomenorrhea, and amenorrhea, reduced luteal phase levels of progesterone, and the consequences of hypoestrogenization which include vaginal dryness, labial atrophy and loss of fat mass of breasts and buttocks in alcoholic women. Indeed, observational studies of endocrine effects of alcoholic beverage abuse by women during the reproductive years have reported an increased prevalence of menstrual dysfunction, and amenorrhea.[118-122] With alcohol abstinence, the amenorrhea may be reversible, whereas with continued abuse the amenorrhea progresses to early menopause.[123] It has further been reported that the ovaries of women dying during their reproductive years of Laennec's cirrhosis have been found to contain no corpora lutea or corpora hemorrhagica, suggesting ovulatory failure for at least several months prior to death.[124]

In contrast to males, acute administration of ethanol to normal women under controlled conditions at specific phases of the menstrual cycle has been reported to produce no consistent effect on levels of either sex steroids or gonadotropins. It has been suggested that such findings are consistent with a hypothesis that a single episode of intoxication is not sufficient to suppress basal hormone levels during either the follicular or luteal phase of the menstrual cycle.[125] It is further possible, given the dynamics of ovarian hormone production vis à vis the phases of follicular maturation, that to disrupt a particular cycle it is necessary that the ethanol insult be delivered at the earliest developmental phase of the particular follicle containing the oocyte destined for ovulation.

Studies in animals have provided data which have replicated the findings of studies in humans describing the effects of chronic abuse of alcoholic beverages on female reproductive function; such animal studies have evaluated ethanol effects on the estrus cycle, on ovulatory function, and on fertility.[36,93,120-139]

In mice, rats and monkeys, it has been demonstrated that as alcohol exposure is prolonged over time or increased in dose, an increased number of female animals show a total loss of estrus cyclicity or a disruption of existing cycles.[125,129-136] Similarly, in rodents and monkeys, an increased incidence of ovulatory failure with ethanol exposure has been documented by findings of absence of ova in the fallopian tubes, absence of ovarian corpora hemorrhagicam and corpora lutea, loss of the midcycle ovulatory gonadotropin surge, and failure of plasma estradiol and progesterone levels to increase in the latter half of the cycle.

That abuse of alcoholic beverages by women during the reproductive years can produce disruption of the menstrual cycle which may result in amenorrhea and ultimately in early menopause has been repeatedly demonstrated in observational clinical studies. Further, such findings have been replicated and extended in various animal models. In spite of such progress, however, the specific mechanisms for the effect of ethanol on the ovarian hypothalamic pituitary axis in general or on follicular maturation and development in particular remain unelucidated.

The Female During the Menopausal Years

As contrasted to women during the reproductive years, postmenopausal women are characterized by a relatively simple pattern of hypothalamic pituitary gonadal axis regulation. By definition, cyclic follicular function has ceased to occur in the menopause; the postmenopausal ovarian stroma, however, continues to produce androgens which are then available for conversion to estrogens at peripheral sites. Although endocrine effects of alcoholic beverage use and abuse in postmenopausal women have been studied to even a lesser degree than such effects in women during the reproductive years, there is a variety of potential pathways by which ethanol may be postulated to influence postmenopausal endocrine function.[137,138] Given that the degree of complexity of hypothalamic pituitary regulation in postmenopausal women is somewhat comparable to that in males, rather than to that in women with reproductive capability, it might be expected that ethanol effects on postmenopausal endocrine function might be readily detectable.

Such is not the case with respect to effects of acute administration of ethanol to normal postmenopausal women. Three recent studies have reported that comparison of the responses following the administration of placebo to responses after ethanol administration has demonstrated no change in circulating levels of either LH or FSH.[127,139,140] These studies in normal postmenopausal women have been confirmed in monkeys. Unfortunately, none of these studies report concomitantly obtained and assayed levels of any steroid hormones and, thus, these reports provide no clue as to acute ethanol effects on postmenopausal levels of androgens or estrogens.

Interestingly, the findings of the few studies of endocrine effects of chronic alcoholic beverage abuse in postmenopausal women with Laennec's cirrhosis echo the observations reported in chronic alcoholic cirrhotic males. None of these four reports is entirely adequate with respect either to sample size and/or to the completeness of the endocrine characterization provided for the postmenopausal women studied; nevertheless these four studies provide generally consistent data: gonadotropins are often decreased while estrogen concentrations are increased.[121,122,141,142]

The question of whether or not moderate consumption of alcoholic beverages by healthy postmenopausal women might increase circulating estrogen has recently been raised. It is known that acute ethanol administration to normal male volunteers results in an increase in the conversion of testosterone to estradiol. It has also been demonstrated in animal studies that even moderate doses of ethanol can stimulate adrenal production of corticosterone, progesterone and androstenedione.[143,144] Given that the major source of estrogens in normal postmenopausal women is the conversion of available androgen precursors to estrogens, and in view of the above findings, it is somewhat surprising that alcoholic beverage consumption has not previously been evaluated as a determinant of circulating levels of estrogens in normal postmenopausal women. The majority of postmenopausal women consume alcoholic beverages to at least a moderate degree.[145-148] Indeed, a recent study in normal postmenopausal women provides evidence that even low to moderate consumption levels of alcohol results in significantly increased circulating concentrations of estradiol.[149-151]

Studies in bilaterally oophorectomized rats have confirmed several of the findings observed in the human studies. Administration of graded doses of alcohol in drinking water (up to 5.5% ethanol) for prolonged periods of time (up to 10 weeks) results in increases in circulating estradiol levels; further, although concentrations of estradiol and LH were significantly correlated in this group of 60 ovariectomized rats, no significant effect of chronic administration of low to moderate doses of ethanol on LH levels was detected.[151]

FEMINIZATION

Androgen and Proandrogen Production

Despite numerous similarities between the sexes in terms of the end stage effects of alcohol abuse on the hypothalamic pituitary gonadal axis, a major difference between alcoholic men and women exists. When one examines the issue of estrogenization, chronic alcoholic women during the reproductive years, like alcoholic men, become progressively hypogonadal with continued alcohol abuse; as a result, they lose their secondary sex characteristics. In contrast, chronic alcoholic men, particularly those with advanced liver disease characterized by portal hypertension and portal systemic shunting, become progressively feminized (hyperestrogenized), as manifested by the physical findings of gynecomastia, palmar erythema, spider angiomata, a female escutcheon and changes in the distribution of body fat and hair, as well as by the biochemical findings of increases in estrogen responsive proteins such as sex steroid binding globulin and neurophysin.

Part of the mechanism responsible for these apparent different responses between the sexes probably reflects the marked difference in normal androgen production rather than the differences in estrogen production rates between the two sexes. For example, primary alcohol-induced gonadal injury in the female reduces estrogen biosynthesis in the female, and androgen biosynthesis in the male. The net result is a clear reduction in plasma estrogen levels in the alcoholic female but markedly reduced testosterone levels in the alcoholic male. As noted earlier, alcohol is a potent inducer of microsomal aromatase activity. Aromatase is the enzyme complex responsible for the conversion of androgens and pro-androgens to estrogens, principally estrone, and to a lesser extent, estradiol. Thus a minor (< 1%) alcohol-associated change in the fraction of proandrogens (androstenedione, dehydroepiandrostrone and dehydroepiandrostrone sulfate) and androgen (testosterone), which are produced in millimolar amounts per day by the male has a profound effect upon estrogen levels which are normally produced in picomolar amounts. Thus despite reduced testicular androgen biosynthesis, the level of plasma estrogens in alcoholic men is either normal (estradiol) or increased (estrone) as a result of a slight increase in the peripheral conversion of androgens to estrogens as a result of alcohol associated aromatase induction.

In the normal female, the production rate of androgens is much lower than in males, and normally a much larger fraction of secreted proandrogens and testosterone are converted to estrogens; thus, a slight increase in the conversion rate of androgens to estrogens as a result of aromatase induction is not sufficient for the maintenance of the female secondary sex characteristics. As a result, alcoholic men become feminized while alcoholic women during the reproductive years become progressively defeminized.

In males, the stimulatory effect of alcohol on adrenal steroid production also contributes directly to the increased circulating levels of estrogens seen in alcoholic cirrhotic males. Not only has adrenal overproduction of weak androgens and estrogen precursors been reported to regularly occur in chronic alcohol men but, also, the adrenals of chronic alcoholic men have been reported to directly produce estrone.[82,152] Specifically, under experimental conditions of adrenal suppression subsequent to gonadal suppression, levels of estrone, estradiol, testosterone and androstenedione are reduced; subsequent gonadal stimulation produces no change in either estrone or androstenedione, while further subsequent adrenal stimulation results in increases in levels of both androstenedione and estrone. Thus, at least in chronic alcoholic males, chronic alcohol stimulation of the adrenals results not only in increased production of the androgen substrate available for conversion, but also in increased direct production of estrone.

The problem of portal systemic shunting which occurs as a consequence of advanced alcoholic liver disease with portal hypertension only compounds the problem of feminization of the male, and it reduces, but does not eliminate the defeminization of the alcoholic woman.[103,152] Specifically as a result of portal systemic shunting of proandrogens (progestens and weak adrenal androgens) large masses of sterols in the millimolar range escape hepatic clearance and are presented to peripheral tissues (fat, muscle, skin, etc.) where alcohol-induced aromatase activity converts a slight but significant fraction to estrogens.

Estrogen Binding Proteins

Yet another factor contributing importantly to the differences between the feminization observed in the male, and the lack of feminization observed in the female, is the effect of alcohol upon cytosolic estrogen binding proteins and receptors.[152-154]

Alcohol increases the level of cytosolic estrogen receptors in both males and females. However, the net change is minimal in the female and marked in the male, principally as a result of the quite different levels observed under basal, nonalcohol abusing, conditions. Moreover, the male is normally protected from estrogen because male hepatocytes contain a cytosolic estrogen binding protein which is not a receptor but which competes for cytosolic estrogen with the receptor. Under normal conditions only 5 or 10% of the cytosolic estrogen binding protein in the male cell is estrogen receptor and the remaining bulk of the estrogen binding protein is nonreceptor protein. Under conditions of alcohol abuse (or feeding of ethanol in animal experiments) the level of estrogen receptor increases slightly, although the level of nonreceptor protein is reduced dramatically. As a consequence, the ratio of receptor to nonreceptor is shifted markedly in favor of the receptor and, as a result, feminization of the male is observed. Such is not the case in the female; estrogen binding in female hepatic cytosol occurs solely via receptors, as the female lacks entirely the male specific nonreceptor estrogen binding protein.

Prolactin and Other Circulating Proteins

Additional factors that may contribute to alcohol-associated gonadal failure are the hyperprolactinemia and the changes in the plasma levels of albumin and sex steroid binding globulin seen in advanced alcoholic liver disease. Chronic alcoholics, particularly those with cirrhosis, have been found to have pituitary prolactin cell hyperplasia at autopsy and some data exist to suggest that prolactin cell secretion may become autonomous in a few alcoholics.[142,155-157] These observations are of interest in that hyperprolactinemia is associated with hypogonadism, as well as deficient gonadotropin secretion and reduced numbers of gonadotropin receptors at the level of the gonad. Equally important is the fact that prolactin may act as a stimulant for adrenal secretion of proandrogens. Such stimulation only enhances the "feminization" of the male and masculinizes the female alcoholic.

Serum albumin is principally responsible for the transport of plasma estrogens, while sex steroid binding globulin is principally responsible for testosterone transport. Chronic alcoholism, as a consequence of malnutrition, liver disease and its various gonadal effects, results in a reduction in plasma albumin levels and a marked increase in the plasma levels of sex steroid binding globulin. The net result for the male is more feminization and less masculinization for any given level of plasma estrogens and androgens. In the case of the female, the net result is a reduction in circulating estrogen levels, probably because less androgen is available for peripheral conversion to estrogen; as a result, progressive defeminization occurs.

Combining the above components of the mechanism responsible for feminization into a unified whole has great appeal. The role of systemic shunting, which would permit steroids to escape the enterohepatic circulation and thus result in increased peripheral tissue exposure, fits well with evidence. Specifically, signs of feminization are seen only in alcoholic males who have developed cirrhosis and the accompanying portal hypertension.[152] Similarly, decreases in hepatic albumin secretion, which would result in increased circulating levels of unbound estrogens, are a common finding in cirrhotics. The reports of alcohol associated decreases in the hepatic male specific nonreceptor estrogen binding protein and concomitant increases in the hepatic content of estrogen receptors provide a mechanism whereby even small increases in circulating levels of estrogen might result in an amplification of estrogen effects. Thus for example, in response to only moderately elevated circulating levels of estrogen which are reported to occur in alcoholic cirrhotic males, the reported increases in sex hormone binding globulin are predictable.

The findings in alcoholics of increases in the adrenal production of weak androgens and pro-androgens, the substrate needed for subsequent conversion to estrogens, along with the findings of increases in the conversion of such precursors to estrogens are consistent with the feminization theory as a whole, but fit the evidence less well. Specifically, while levels of estrone in cirrhotic alcoholic males have consistently been reported to be elevated significantly, the levels of the five times more potent estrogen, estradiol, have been reported to be somewhat increased but not significantly different from levels in normal controls.[77-79,93,94,158] Given the degree of hyperestrogenization observed in feminized alcoholic cirrhotic males, perhaps it is possible that such men are exposed not only to the steroidal estrogens such as estrone and estradiol, but also to nonsteroidal estrogens as well. In passing, it is worth noting that if nonsteroidal estrogens were present, they would not be detected by a radioimmunoassay in which the antibody recognizes estrone or estradiol but does not cross-react with nonsteroidal estrogenic substances.

Nonsteroidal Estrogens

Very recent reports provide data that fit a hypothesis which includes not only all of the components of the feminization mechanism discussed above, but which also incorporates exposure to biologically active nonsteroidal estrogens as well. Specifically, recent studies provide evidence that bourbon, a whiskey made from corn, contains the biologically active nonsteroidal phytoestrogen biochanin A.[159,160,161] In addition to isolating and identifying this estrogen of plant origin in an extract of bourbon, these reports also demonstrate that the bourbon concentrate not only produces two measurable estrogenic dose responses in an appropriate animal model but also interacts with estrogen receptors in a dose dependent manner. Although it yet remains to be demonstrated that other alcoholic beverages contain biologically active phytoestrogens, these reports suggest, at the very least, that the mechanisms responsible for the feminization observed in some alcoholic cirrhotic men have not yet been fully elucidated.

REFERENCES

1. Cohen, S. (1700) The pharmacology of alcohol. *Postgrad Med* 64:97-102.

2. Mezey, E. (1976) Ethanol metabolism and drug interactions. *Biochem Pharmacol* 25:869-875.

3. Datta, S., Hay, V.M. and Pleuvry, B.J. (1974) Effects of pregnancy and associated hormones in mouse intestine *in vivo* and *in vitro*. *Pfluegers Arch* 346:87-93.

4. Cripps, A.W. and Williams, V.J. (1975) The effect of pregnancy and lactation on food intake, gastrointestinal anatomy and the absorptive capacity of the small intestine in the albino rat. *Br J Nutr* 33:17-25.

5. Van Thiel, D.H., Gavaler, J.S. and Stremple, J.F. (1979) Lower esophageal sphincter pressure during the normal menstrual cycle. *Am J Obstet Gynecol* 134:64-69.

6. Van Thiel, D.H., Gavaler, J.S. and Stremple, J.F. (1976) Lower esophageal sphincter pressure in women using sequential oral contraceptives. *Gastroenterology* 71:232-241.

7. Van Thiel, D.H., Gavaler, J.S. and Joshi, S.H. (1977) Heartburn of pregnancy. *Gastroenterology* 72:666-671.

8. Scott, L.D., Lester, R. and Van Thiel, D.H. (1983) Pregnancy related changes in small intestinal myoelectric activity in the rat. *Gastroenterology* 84:301-307.

9. Wald, A., Van Thiel, D.H. and Hoechstetter, L. (1982) Effect of pregnancy on gastrointestinal transit. *Digestive Disease and Sci* 27:1015-1018.

10. Feinman, L., Baraona, E., Matsuzaki, S., Korsten, M. and Lieber, C.S. (1978) Concentration dependence of ethanol metabolism *in vivo* in rats and man. *Alcoholism Clin Exp Res* 2:381-385.

11. Grunnet, N., Quistorff, B. and Thieden, H.I.D. (1973) Rate limiting factors in ethanol oxidation by isolated rat parenchymal cells: effect of ethanol concentration, fructose, pruvate and pyrazole. *Eur J Biochem* 40:275-282.

12. Matsuzaki, S., Gordon, E. and Lieber, C.S. (1981) Increased alcohol dehydrogenase independent ethanol oxidation at high ethanol concentrations in isolated rat hepatocytes: the effect of chronic ethanol feeding. *J Pharmacol Exp Ther* 217:133-137.

13. Teschke, R., Hasumura, Y. and Lieber, C.S. (1976) Hepatic ethanol metabolism: respective roles of alcohol dehydrogenase, the microsomal ethanol oxidizing system and catalase. *Arch Biochem Biophys* 175:635-643.

14. Aschenasy-Lehr, P. (1958) Action d'un oestrogene sur la consommation spontance d'un boisson alcoolisee chez de rat. *Seanc Acad Sci Paris* 247:1044-1047.

15. Aschenasy-Lehr, P. (1960) Action inhibitrice d'un hormone oestorgene sur la consommation spontance d'alcool parle rat. *Revue Fr. Etud. Clin Biol* 5:132-138.

16. Mardones, J. (1960) Experimentally induced changes in the free selection of ethanol. *Int Rev Neurobiol* 2:41-76.

17. Emerson, G.A., Brown, R.C., Nash, J.B. and Moore, W.T. (1952) Species variation in preference for alcohol and in effects of diet or drugs on this preference. *J Pharmacol Exp Ther* 106:384-388.

18. Ericksson, K. (1969) Effects of ovariectomy and contraceptive hormones on voluntary alcohol consumption in the albino rat. *Jap J Alcohol Stud* 4:1-5.

19. Little, R.E., Schultz, F.A. and Mandell, W. (1976) Drinking during pregnancy. *J Stud Alcohol* 37:375-379.

20. Little, R.E. and Streissguth, A.P. (1978) Drinking during pregnancy in alcoholic women. *Alcohol Clin Exp Res* 2:179-183.

21. Zeiner, A.R. and Kegg, P.S. (1980) Menstrual cycle and oral contraceptive effects on alcohol pharmacokinetics in caucasian females. *Alcohol Clin Exp Res* 4:233-238.

22. Zeiner, A.R. and Kegg, P.S. (1981) Menstrual cycle and oral contraceptive effects on alcohol pharmacokinetics in caucasian females. *Curr Alcohol* 8:325-328.

23. Zeiner, A.R. and Kegg, P.S. (1981) Effects of sex steroids on ethanol pharmacokinetics and autonomic reactivity. *Prog Biochem Pharmacol* 18:130-142.

24. Jones, B.M. and Jones, M.K. (1976) Alcohol effects in women during the menstrual cycle. *Ann NY Acad Sci* 272:576-587.

25. Jones, B.M. and Jones, M.K. (1976) Women and alcohol: Intoxication metabolism and the menstrual cycle, In: *Alcoholism Problems in Women and Children*, p. 103. Greenblatt, M. and Schuckt, M.A. (eds), Grune and Stratton, New York.

26. Jones, B.M. and Jones, M.K. (1977) Interaction of alcohol, oral contraceptives and menstrual cycle with stimulus response compatibility. In: *Currents in Alcoholism*, Vol II, Psychiatric, Psychological Social and Epidemiological Studies. p 457 Seixas, F.A. (ed) Grune & Stratton, New York.

27. Jones, B.M., Jones, M.K. and Paredes, A. (1976) Oral contraceptives and ethanol metabolism. *Revta Invest Clin Mexico* 24:95-99.

28. Marshall, A.W., Kingstone, D., Boss, M. and Morgan, M.Y. (1983) Ethanol elimination in males and females relationship to menstrual cycle and body composition. *Hepatology* 3:701-706.

29. Dubowski, K.M. (1976) Human pharmacokinetics of ethanol: I peak

blood concentrations and elimination in male and female subjects. *Alcohol Technical Reports*, Oklahoma City 5:55-63.

30. Brick, J., Nathan, P.E., Wentrick, E., Frankenstein, W. and Shapiro, A. (1986) The effect of menstrual cycle on blood alcohol levels and behavior. *J Stud Alcohol* 47:472-477.

31. Goist, K.C. Jr. and Sutker, P.B. (1985) Acute alcohol intoxication and body composition in women and men. *Pharmacol Biochem Behav* 22:811-814.

32. Jones, M.K. and Jones, B.M. (1984) Ethanol metabolism in women taking oral contraceptives. *Alcoholism Clin Exp Res* 8:24-28.

33. Mello, N.K., Brec, M.P., Skupny, A.S.T. and Mendelson, J. (1984) Blood alcohol levels as a function of menstrual cycle phase in female Macaque monkeys. *Alcohol* 1:27-31.

34. Ghatcher, E.M., Jones, B.M. and Jones, M.K. (1977) Cognitive deficits in alcoholic women. *Alcohol Clin Exp Res* 1:371-377.

35. Jones, B.M., Jones, M.K. and Hatcher, E.M. (1980) Cognitive deficits in women alcoholics as a function of gynecological status. *J Stud Alcohol* 41:140-146.

36. Linnoila, M., Erwin, C.W., Ramm, D., Cleveland, W.P. and Brendle, A. (19809) Effects of alcohol on psychomotor performance of women: interaction with menstrual cycle. *Alcohol Clin Exp Res* 4:302-305.

37. Goldberg, L. and Stortebecker, T.P. (1943) The antinarcotic effect of estrone on alcohol intoxication. *Acta Phys Scandinav* 5:289-296.

38. Fabian, M., Hoehla, N., Silberstein, J. and Parsons, O.A. (1980) Menstrual states and neuropsychological functioning. *Biol Psychol Bull* 6:37-45.

39. Hay, W.M., Nathan, P.E., Heermans, H.W. and Frankenstein, W. (1984) Menstrual cycle tolerance and blood alcohol level discrimination ability. *Addict Behav* 9:67-77.

40. Sutker, P.G., Libet, J.M., Allain, A.N. and Randall, C.L. (1983) Alcohol use, negative mood states, and menstrual cycle phases. *Alcoholism: Clinical and Experimental Research* 7:327-331.

41. Rachamin, G., MacDonald, J.A., Walid, S., Clapp, J.J., Khann, J.M. and Israel, Y. (1980) Modulation of alcohol dehydrogenase and ethanol metabolism by sex hormones in the spontaneously hypertensive rat. *Biochem J* 186:484-490.

42. Mezey, E. and Potter, J.J. (1982) Effect of dihydrotestosterone on rat liver alcohol dehydrogenase activity. *Hepatology* 2:359-365.

43. Mezey, E., Potter, J.J. and Tsitouras, P.D. (1981) Liver alcohol dehydrogenase activity in the female rat: effects of ovariectomy and estradiol administration. *Life Sci* 29:1171-1176.

44. Mezey, E., Potter, J.J. and Diehl, A.M. (1986) Depression of alcohol dehydrogenase activity in rat hepatocyte culture by dihydrotestosterone. *Biochem Pharmacol* 35:335-339.

45. Hamerick, M.E., Zampaglione, N.G., Stripp, B. and Gillette, S.R. (1973) Investigation of the effects of methyltestosterone, cortisone, and spirono-

lactone on the hepatic microsomal mixed function oxidase system in male and female rats. *Biochem Pharmac* 22:293-310.

46. Kato, R. and Gillette, J.R. (1965) Sex differences in the effects of abnormal physiological states on the metabolism of drugs by rat liver microsomes. *J Pharmacol Exp Ther* 150:285-291.

47. Schenkmann, J.B., Frey, I., Remmer, H. and Estrabrook, R.W. (1967) Sex differences in drug metabolism by rat liver. *Molec Pharmacol* 3:516-525.

48. Einarsson, K., Gustafsson, J.A., Sjovall, J. and Zietz, E. (1975) Dose dependent effects of ethinyloestradiol, diethylstillbesterol and oestradiol on the metabolism of 4-androstene-3, 17-dione in rate microsomes. *Acta Endocrinol* (Copenh) 78:54-64.

49. Eagon, P.K., Porter, L.E., Francavilla, A., DiLeo, A. and Van Thiel, D.H. (1985) Estrogen and androgen receptors in liver: Their role in liver disease and regeneration. *Seminars in Liver Disease* 5:59-69.

50. O'Malley, K., Stevenson, I.H. and Crooks, J. (1972) Impairment of human drug metabolism by oral contraceptive steroids. *Clin Pharmacol Ther* 13:552-557.

51. Crawford, J.S. and Rudofsky, S. (1966) Some alterations in the pattern of drug metabolism associated with pregnancy, oral contraceptives and the newly born. *Br J Anaesth* 38:445-454.

52. Kling, O.R. and Christensen, H.D. (1979) Caffeine elimination in late pregnancy. *Fed Proc* 38:266-269.

53. Patwardhan, R.V., Desmond, P.V., Johnson, R.F. and Schenker, S. (1980) Impaired elimination of caffeine by oral contraceptives. *J Lab Clin Med* 95:603-608.

54. Teschke, R. and Heymann, K. (1982) Effect of sex hormones on the activities of hepatic alcohol metabolizing enzymes in male rats. *Enzyme* 28:268-277.

55. Cicero, J.J., Bernard, J.D. and Newman, K. (1980) Effects of castration and chronic morphine administration on liver alcohol dehydrogenase and the metabolism of ethanol in the male Sprague Dawley rat. *J Pharmacol Exp Ther* 215:317-324.

56. Joliffe, N. and Jellinek, E.M. (1941) Vitamin deficiencies and liver cirrhosis. Part VII cirrhosis of the liver. *Q J Stud Alcohol* 2:544-583.

57. Terris, M. (1967) Epidemiology of cirrhosis of the liver, national mortality data. *Am J Public Health* 57:2076-2080.

58. Whitlock, F.A. (1974) Liver cirrhosis, alcoholism and alcohol consumption. *Q J Stud Alcohol* 35:588-605.

59. Schmidt, W. (1975) Disagreement in experimental, clinical and epidemiological evidence on the etiology of alcohol cirrhosis. In: *Alcohol Liver Pathology* Khanna, J.M., Israel, Y. and Kalsrt, H. (eds) p 106 Addition Research Foundation, Toronto.

60. Lelbach, W.K. (1975) Quantitative aspects of drinking in alcoholic liver disease. In: *Alcohol Liver Pathology* Khanna, J.M., Israel, Y. and Kalant, H. (eds) p 320 Addition Research Foundation, Toronto.

61. Wilkinson, P., Santamaria, J.N. and Rankin, J.G. (1969) Epidemiology of alcoholic cirrhosis. *Australian Ann Med* 18:222-226.

62. Wilkinson, P., Kornaczewski, A., Rankin, J.G. and Santamaria, J.N. (1971) Physical disease in alcoholism: initial survey of 1000 patients. *Med J Aust* 1:1217-1225.

63. Gavaler, J.S. (1982) Sex related differences in ethanol induced liver disease: Antifactural or real? *Alcoholism Clin Exp Res* 6:186-196.

64. Bhattacharyya, D.N. and Rake, M.O. (1983) Correlation of alcohol consumption with liver damage in men and women. *Alcohol and Alcoholism* 18:181-184.

65. Krasner, N., Davis, M., Portmann, B. and Williams, R. (1977) Changing patterns of alcoholic liver disease in Great Britain: relation to sex and signs of autoimmunity. *Brit Med J* 1:1497-1500.

66. Pares, A., Calballeria, J., Bruguera, M., Torres, M. and Rodes, J. (1986) Histological course of alcoholic hepatitis: influence of abstinence, sex and extent of hepatic damage. *J Hepatology* 2:33-42.

67. Saunders, J.B., Davies, M. and Williams, R. (1981) Do women develop alcoholic liver disease more readily than men. *Brit Med J* 282:1140-1143.

68. Bruix, J., Bruguera, M. and Bordas, J. (1981) Hepatitis alcoholico estudio comparativo en varones y mujeres *Gastroenterol Hepatol* 4:341-344.

69. Morgan, M.Y. and Sherlock, S. (1977) Sex related differences among 100 patients with alcoholic liver disease. *Brit Med J* 1:935-941.

70. Spain, D.M. (1945) Portal cirrhosis of the liver: a review of 250 necropsies with reference to sex differences. *Am J Clin Pathol* 15:215-218.

71. Peguignot, G., Chabert, C., Eydoux, H. and Courcoul, M.A. (1974) tation du risque de cirrhose en fonction de la ration d'alcool. *Revue Alcoholism* 20:191-202.

72. Lloyd, C.W. and Williams, R.H., (1948) Endocrine changes associated with Laennec's cirrhosis of the liver. *Am. J. Med* 4:315-320.

73. Chopra, I.J., Tulchinsky, D. and Greenway, F.L. (1973) Estrogen-androgen imbalance in hepatic cirrhosis. *Ann Intern Med* 79:198-203.

74. Galvao-Teles, A., Anderson, D.C., Burke, C.W., Marshall, J.C., Corker, C.S., Brown, R.L. and Clark, J.L. (1973) Biologically active androgens and oestradiol in men with chronic liver disease. *Lancet* 1:173-178.

75. Kent, J.R., Scaramuzzi, R.J., Lauwers, W., Parlow, A.F., Hill, M., Penardi, R. and Hilliard, J. (1973) Plasma testosterone, estradiol and gonadotropin in hepatic insufficiency. *Gastroenterology* 64:111-116.

76. Gordon, G.G., Olivo, J., Raffi, F. and Southren, A.L. (1975) Conversion of androgens to estrogens in cirrhosis of the liver. *J Clin Endocrinol Metab* 40:1018-1023.

77. Kley, H.K., Nieschlag, E., Wiegelmann, W., Solbach, M.G. and Kruskemper, H.L. (1975) Steroid hormones and their binding in plasma of male patients with fatty liver, chronic hepatitis and liver cirrhosis. *Acta. Endocrinol* 79:275-280.

78. Van Thiel, D.H., Gavaler, J.S., Lester, R., Loriaux, D.L. and Braun-

stein, G.D. (1975b) Plasma estrone, prolactin, neurophysin, and sex steroid binding protein in chronic alcoholic men. *Metabolism* 24:1015-1019.

79. Baker, H.W.G., Burger, H.G., Dekretser, D.M., Dulmanis, A., Hudson, B., O'Connor, S., Paulsen, C.A., Purcell, N., Rennie, G.C., Seah, C.S., Taft, H.P. and Wang, C. (1976) A study of the endocrine manifestations of hepatic cirrhosis. *Quart J Med* 45:145-165.

80. Lindholm, J., Fabricius-Bjerre, N., Bahnsen, M., Boiesen, P., Hagen, C. and Christensen, T. (1978) Sex steroids and sex-steroid binding globulin in males with chronic alcoholism. *Euro J Clin Invest* 8:273-278.

81. Van Thiel, D.H., Lester, R. and Vaitukaitis, J. (1978a) Evidence for a defect in pituitary secretion of luteinizing hormone in chronic alcoholic men. *J Clin Endocrinol Metab* 47:499-507.

82. Van Thiel, D.H. and Loriaux, D.L. (1979c) Evidence for an adrenal origin of plasma estrogens in alcoholic men. *Metabolism* 28:536-541.

83. Badr, F.M. and Bartke, A. (1974) Effect of ethyl alcohol on plasma testosterone levels in mice. *Steroids* 23:921-926.

84. Cicero, T.J. and Badger, T.M. (1977) Effects of alcohol on the hypothalamic pituitary gonadal axis in the male rat. *J Pharm Exp Ther* 201:427-432.

85. Cicero, T.J., Bernstein, D. and Badger, T.M. (1975) Effects of acute alcohol administration on reproductive endocrinology in the male rat. *Alcoholism: Clin Exp Res* 2:249-255.

86. Cicero, T.J. and Bell, R.D. (1980) Effects of ethanol and acetaldehyde on the biosynthesis of testosterone in the rodent testes. *Biochem Biophy Res Comm* 94:814-819.

87. Cicero, T.J. and Bell, R.D. (1980) Acetaldehyde directly inhibits the conversion of androstenedione to testosterone. In: *Alcohol and Acetaldehyde Metabolizing Systems*, Vol. 4., pp 346-353 Thurman, R.G. (ed) Plenum, New York.

88. Cicero, T.J., Bell, R.D., Meyer, E.R. and Badger, T.M. (1980) Ethanol and acetaldehyde directly inhibit testicular steroidogenesis. *J Pharmacol Exp Ther* 213:228-233.

89. Cicero, T.J., Newman, K.S. and Meyer, E.R. (1981) Ethanol induced inhibitions of testicular steroidogenesis in the male rat: mechanisms of action. *Life Sci* 28:871-877.

90. Van Thiel, D.H., Gavaler, J.S., Lester, R. and Goodman, M.D. (1975) Alcohol-induced testicular atrophy: an experimental model for hypogonadism occurring in chronic alcoholic men. *Gastroenterology* 69:326-332.

91. Van Thiel, D.H., Gaveler, J.S., Cobb, C.F., Sherins, R. and Lester, R. (1979) Alcohol-induced testicular atrophy in the adult male rat. *Endocrinology* 105:888-895.

92. Badr, F.M., Bartke, A., Dalterio, S. and Bugler, W. (1977) Suppression of testosterone production by ethyl alcohol: possible mode of action. *Steroids* 30:647-657.

93. Gavaler, J.S., Van Thiel, D.H. and Lester, R. (1980) Ethanol, a gonadal toxin in the mature rat of both sexes: similarities and differences. *Alcoholism: Clin Exp Res* 4:271-276.

94. Van Thiel, D.H., Gavaler, J.S., Spero, J.A., Egler, K.M., Wight, C., Sanghvi, A., Hasiba, U. and Lewis, J.H. (1981b) Patterns of hypothalamic-pituitary-gonadal dysfunction in men with liver disease due to differing etiologies. *Hepatology* 1:39-46.

95. Mendelson, J.H., Mello, N.K. and Ellingboe, J. (1977) Effects of acute alcohol intake on pituitary gonadal hormones in normal human males. *J Pharmacol Exp Ther* 202:676-681.

96. Ylikahri, R., Huttunen, I.M., Harkonen, M., Seuderling, U., Onikki, S., Karonen, S.I. and Aldercreutz, H. (1974) Low plasma testosterone values in men during hangover. *J Steroid Biochem* 5:655-662.

97. Gordon, G.G., Altman, K., Southren, A.L., Rubin, E. and Lieber, C.S. (1976) Effect of alcohol (ethanol) administration on sex hormone metabolism in men. *N Eng J Med* 295:793-798.

98. Van Thiel, D.H. (1983) Ethanol: its adverse effects upon the hypothalamic pituitary gonadal axis. *J Lab Clin Med* 101:21-33.

99. Cobb, C.F., Ennis, M.F., Van Thiel, D.H., Gavaler, J.S. and Lester, R. (1980) Isolated testes perfusion: a method using a cell- and protein-free perfusate useful for the evaluation of potential drug and/or metabolic injury. *Metabolism* 30:71-79.

100. Van Thiel, D.H., Gavaler, J.S., Cobb, C.F., Santucci, L. and Graham, T.O. (1983) Ethanol, a Leydig cell toxin: evidence obtained *in vivo* and *in vitro*. *Pharmacol Biochem Behav* 18:317-323.

101. Santucci, L., Graham, T.O. and Van Thiel, D.H. (1983) Inhibition of testosterone production by rat Leydig cells with ethanol and acetaldehyde: prevention of ethanol toxicity with 4-methylpyrazol. *Alcoholism: Clin Exp Res* 7:135-139.

102. Gavaler, J.S., Gay, V., Egler, K.M. and Van Thiel, D.H. (1983) Evaluation of the differential *in vivo* toxic effects of ethanol and acetaldehyde on the hypothalamic-pituitary-gonadal axis using 4-methylpyrazole. *Alcoholism: Clin Exp Res* 7:332-336.

103. Van Thiel, D.H., Gavaler, J.S., Slone, F.L., Cobb, C.F., Smith Jr., W.I., Bron, K.M. and Lester, R. (1980) Is feminization in alcoholic men due in part to portal hypertension: a rat model. *Gastroenterology* 78:81-91.

104. Van Thiel, D.H., Cobb, C.F., Herman, G.B., Perez, H.A., Estes, L. and Gavaler, J.S. (1981a) An examination of various mechanisms for ethanol-induced testicular injury: studies utilizing the isolated perfused rat testes. *Endocrinology* 109:2009-2015.

105. Gavaler, J.S., Perez, H.A., Estes, L. and Van Thiel, D.H. (1983) Morphologic alterations of rat Leydig cells induced by ethanol. *Pharmacol Biochem Behav* 18:341-347.

106. Gordon, G.G., Southren, A.L. and Lieber, C.S. (1979) Hypogonadism and feminization in the male: A triple effect of alcohol. *Alcoholism: Clin Exp Res* 3:210-216.

107. Gordon, G.G., Southren, A.L., Vittek, J. and Lieber, C.S. (1979) The

effect of alcohol ingestion on hepatic aromatase activity and plasma steroid hormones in the rat. *Metabolism* 28:20-27.

108. Ellingboe, J. and Varanelli, C.C. (1979) Ethanol inhibits testosterone biosynthesis by direct action on Leydig cells. *Res Comm Chem Pathol Pharmacol* 28:87-92.

109. Johnston, D.E., Chiao, Y-B., Gavaler, J.S. and Van Thiel, D.H. (1981) Inhibition of testosterone synthesis by ethanol and acetaldehyde. *Biochem Pharmacol* 30:1827.

110. Chiao, Y-B., Johnston, D.E., Gavaler, J.S. and Van Thiel, D.H. (1981) Effect of chronic ethanol feeding on testicular content of enzymes required for testosteronogenesis. *Alcoholism: Clin Exp Res* 5:230-238.

111. Gordon, G.G., Vittek, J., Southren, A.L., Munnang, P. and Lieber, C.S. (1980) Effect of chronic alcohol ingestion on the biosynthesis of steroids in rat testicular homogenates in vitro. *Endocrinology* 106:1880-1886.

112. Messiha, F.S. (1981) Subcellular fractionation of alcohol and aldehyde dehydrogenase in the rat testicle. *Prog Biochem Pharmacol* 18:155-160.

113. Van Thiel, D.H., Gavaler, J.S. and Lester, R. (1974) Ethanol inhibition of vitamin A in the testes: possible mechanism for sterility in alcoholics, *Science* 186:941-942.

114. Chiao, Y-B. and Van Thiel, D.H. (1983) Biochemical mechanisms that contribute to alcohol-induced hypogonadism in the male. *Alcoholism: Clin Exp Res* 7:131-138.

115. Chaio, Y-B. and Van Thiel, D.H. (1986) Characterization of rat testicular alcohol dehydrogenase. *Alcohol Alcoholism* 21:9-15.

116. Rosenblum, E.R., Gavaler, J.S. and Van Thiel, D.H. (1985) Lipid peroxidation: a mechanism for ethanol associated testicular injury in rats. *Endocrinology* 116:311-318.

117. rosenblum, E.R., Gavaler, J.S. and Van Thiel, D.H. (1987) Vitamin A at pharmacologic doses ameliorates the membrane lipid peroxidation injury and testicular atrophy which occur with chronic ethanol feeding in rats. *Alcohol Alcoholism* 22:241-249.

118. Moskovic, S (1975) Effect of chronic alcohol intoxication on ovarian dysfunction. *STIAR* 20:2-5.

119. Jones-Saumty, D.J., Fabian, M.S. and Parsons, D.A. (1981) Medical status and cognitive functioning in alcoholic women. *Alcoholism: Clin Exp Res* 5:372-377.

120. Hugues, J.N., Perret, G., Adessi, G., Coste, T. and Modigliani, E. (1978) Effect of chronic alcoholism on the pituitary gonadal function of women during menopausal transition and in the postmenopausal period. *Biomedicine* 29:279-286.

121. Hugues, J.N., Coste, T., Perret, G., Jayle, M.F., Sebaqun, J. and Modigliani, E. (1980) Hypothalamic pituitary ovarian function in thirty-one women with chronic alcoholism. *clin Endocrinol* 12:543-548.

122. Wilsnack, S.C., Klassen, A.D. and Wilsnack, R.W. (1984) Drinking

and reproductive dysfunction among women in a 1982 national survey. *Alcoholism: Clin Exp Res* 8:451-456.

123. Ryback, R.S. (1977) Chronic alcohol consumption and menstruation. *J Am Med Assoc* 238:2143-2149.

124. Jung, Y. and Russfield, A.B. (1972) Prolactin cells in the hypophysis of cirrhotic patients. *Arch Pathol* 94:265-271.

125. McNamee, B., Grant, J., Ratcliffe, J., Ratcliffe, W. and Oliver, J. (1979) Lack of effect of alcohol on pituitary gonadal hormones in women. *Br J Addict* 74:316-321.

126. Mendelson, J.H., Mello, N.K., Barli, S., Ellingboe, J., Bree, M., Harvey, K., King, N. and Seghal, R. (1983) Ethanol Tolerance and Dependence: Endocrinologic Aspects Alcohol effects on female reproductive hormones. Cicero, T.J., (ed) *NIAAA Research p 1299 Monograph*, Washington, D.C., (DHHS Pub. No. (ADM) 83-1285).

127. Mendelson, J.H., Mello, N.K. and Ellingboe, J.H. (1981) acute alcohol intake and pituitary gonadal hormones in normal human females. *J Pharmacol Exp Ther* 218:23-28.

128. Valimaki, M., Harkonen, M. and Ylikahri, R. (1983) Acute effects of alcohol on female sex hormones. *Alcoholism: Clin Exp Res* 7:289-294.

129. Cranston, E.M. (1958) Effect of tranquilizers and other agents on the sexual cycle of mice. *Proc Soc Exp Biol Med* 98:320-328.

130. Aron, E., Flanzy, M., Combescot, C., Puisais, J., Demaret, J., Reynouard-Brault, F. and Igbert, C. (1965) 7L'alcool est-il dans le vin l'element qui perturbe chez la ratte le cycle vaginal? *Bull Acad Natl Med* 149:112-118.

131. Kieffer, J.D. and Ketchel, M. (1970) Blockade of ovulation in the rat by ethanol. *Acta Endocrinol* 65:117-123.

132. Van Thiel, D.H., Gavaler, J.S., Sherins, R.J. and Lester, R. (1977) Alcohol-induced ovarian failure in the rat. *J Clin Invest* 61:624-632.

133. Eskay, R.L., Ryback, R.S., Goodman, M. and Majchrowicz, E. (1982) Effect of chronic ethanol administration on plasma levels of LH and the estrus cycle in the female rat. *Alcoholism: Clin Exp Res* 5:204-210.

134. Bo, W.J., Krueger, W.A., Rudeen, P.K. and Symmes, S.K., (1982) Ethanol-induced alterations in the morphology and function of the rat ovary. *Anat Rec* 202:255-260.

135. Mello, N.K., Bree, M.P., Mendelson, J.H. and Ellingboe, J. (1983) Alcohol self-administration disrupts reproductive function in female Macaque monkeys. *Science* 211:677-680.

136. Chaudhury, R.R. and Matthews, M. (1966) Effects of alcohol on the fertility of female rabbits. *J Endocrinol* 34:275-280.

137. Blake, C.A. (1978) Paradoxical effects of drugs acting on the central nervous system on the preovulatory release of pituitary luteinizing hormone in pro-oestrous rats. *J Endocrinol* 79:319-325.

138. Gavaler, J.S. (1983) Sex related differences in ethanol induced hypogonadism and sex steroid responsive tissue atrophy: analysis of the weanling ethanol-fed rat model using epidemiologic methods. In: *Ethanol Tolerance and Depen-*

dence: Endocrinologic Aspects. Cicero, T.J., (ed) NIAAA Research Monograph No 13 Washington, D.C., (DHHS Pub. No. (ADM) 83-1258).

139. Mendelson, J.H., Mello, N.K., Ellingboe, J. and Bavli, S., (1985) Alcohol effects on plasma luteinizing hormone levels in postmenopausal women. *Pharmacol Biochem. Behav* 22:233-240.

140. Valimaki, M., Penkonen, K. and Ylikahri, R. Acute ethanol intoxication does not influence gonadotropin secretion in postmenopausal women. *Alcohol Alcoholism* in press.

141. Valimaki, M., Penkonen, K., Salaspuro, M., Harkonen, M., Hirvonen, E. and Ylikahri, R. (1984) Sex hormones in amenorrheic women with alcoholic liver disease. *J Clin Endocrinol Metab* 59:133-139.

142. Clark, W.B. and Widanik, L. (1982) Alcohol use and alcohol problems among U.S. adults: results of the 1979 national survey, In *Alcohol Consumption and Related Problems*, NIAAA Alcohol and Health Monograph No. 1, Washington, D.C., (DHHS Pub.; No. (ADM) 82-1190) pg 3.

143. Cobb, C.F., Van Thiel, D.H., Gavaler, J.S. and Lester, R. (1981) Effects of ethanol and acetaldehyde on the rat adrenal. *Metabolism* 30:537-543.

144. Cobb, C.F., Van Thiel, D.H. and Gavaler, J.S. (1981) Isolated rat adrenal perfusion: a new method to study adrenal function. *J Surg Res* 31:347-353.

145. Goodwin, J.S., Sanchez, C.J., Thomas, P., Hunt, C., Garry, P.J. and Goodwin, J.M. (1987) Alcohol intake in a healthy elderly population. *Am J Public Health* 77:173-179.

146. Wechsler, H. (1980) Summary of the literature: epidemiology of male and female drinking over the last century, in Alcoholism and Alcohol Abuse Among Women, p 841 *NIAAA Research Monograph No. 1*, WAshington, D.C., (DHEW Pub. No. (ADM) 80-835) 3.

147. Graham, K. (1986) Identifying and measuring alcohol abuse among the elderly: serious problems with instrumentation. *J Stud Alc* 47:322-327.

148. Gomberg, E.S.L. (1982) Alcohol use and alcohol problems among the elderly. In *Special Population issues*, NIAAA Alcohol and Health Monograph No. 4, Washington, D.C., (DHHS Pub. No. (ADM) 82-1193) 263.

149. Gavaler, J.S., Belle, S. and Cauley, J. Effects of moderate alcoholic beverage consumption on estradiol levels in normal postmenopausal women. *Alcoholism: Clin Exp Res* in press.

150. Gavaler, J.S. and Rosenblum, E.R. (1987) Exposure dependent effects of ethanol administered in drinking water on serum estradiol and uterus mass in sexually mature oophorectomized rats: a rat model for bilaterally ovariectomized/postmenopausal women. *J Stud Alc* 48:295-303.

151. Van Thiel, D.H., Rosenblum, E.R., Pohl, C. and Gavaler, J.S. (1985) Lack of an effect of ethanol administered in drinking water to sexually mature oophorectomized rats on LH levels. *Alcoholism: Clin Exp Res* 9:194.

152. Van Thiel, D.H. (1979) Feminization of chronic alcoholic men: a formulation. *Yale J Biol Med* 52:219-255.

153. Eagon, P.K., Porter, L.E., Gavaler, J.S., Egler, K.M. and Van Thiel, D.H. (1981) Effect of ethanol feeding upon levels of a male-specific hepatic estro-

gen binding protein: a possible mechanism for feminization. *Alcoholism: Clin Exp Res* 5:183-187.

154. Eagon, P.K., Zdunek, R.J., Van Thiel, D.H., Singletary, B., Egler, K. Gavaler, J.S. and Porter, L.E. (1981) Alcohol-induced changes in hepatic estrogen binding proteins. *Arch Biochem Biophys* 210:48-54.

155. Van Thiel, D.H., McClain, C.J., Elson, M.K. and McMillan, M.J. (1978b) Hyperprolactinemia and thyrotropin releasing factor (TRH) responses in men with alcoholic liver disease. *Alcoholism: Clin Exp Res* 2:344-348.

156. Van Thiel, D.H., McClain, C.J., Elson, M.K., McMillin, M.J. and Lester, R. (1978) Evidence for autonomous secretion of prolactin in some alcoholic men with cirrhosis and gynecomastia. *Metabolism* 27:1178-1184.

157. Tarquini, B., Gheri, R. and Anichini, P. (1977) Circadran study of immunoreactive prolactin in patients with cirrhosis of the liver. *Gastroenterology* 73:116-121.

158. Pentikainen, P.J., Pentikainen, L.A., Azarnoff, D.L. and Dujovne, C.A. (1975) Plasma levels and excretion of estrogens in urine in chronic liver disease. *Gastroenterology* 69:20-26.

159. Gavaler, J.S., Imhoff, A.F., Pohl, C.R., Rosenblum, E.R. and Van Thiel, D.H. (1987) Alcoholic beverages: a source of estrogenic substances? In: *Advances in Biomedical Alcohol Research* pp 545-549. Lindros, K.O., Ylikahri, R. and Kiianmaa, K., (eds) Pergamon Press, Oxford.

160. Rosenblum, E.R., Van Thiel, D.H., Campbell, I.M., Eagon, P.K. and Gavaler, J.S. (1987) Separation and identification of phyto-estrogenic compounds isolated from bourbon. In: *Advances in Biomedical Alcohol Research* Lindros, K.O., Ylikahri, R. and Kiianmaa, K. (eds) pp 551-555, Pergamon Press, Oxford.

161. Gavaler, J.S., Rosenblum, E.R., Van Thiel, D.H., Eagon, P.K., Pohl, C.R., Campbell, I.M. and Gavaler, J. Biologically active phyto-estrogens are present in bourbon. *Alcoholism: Clin Exp Res* in press.

Review of the Molecular Biology of the Human Alcohol Dehydrogenase Genes and Gene Products

Robin W. Cotton, PhD
David Goldman, MD

SUMMARY. Using protein and enzymatic methods, a major role in ethanol metabolism was assigned to the alcohol dehydrogenase (ADH) enzymes. Three major classes of ADHs were described on the basis of structure and function, including timing and location of expression. Polymorphic variants, including a common functional variant, were identified. Molecular cloning allowed the demonstration of a high degree of sequence homology between the three class I ADH genes and enabled the definition of ADH variants at the DNA sequence level. The existence of an ADH gene cluster on chromosome 4 and the shared evolutionary roots of these genes suggests that the continued integration of studies of the different ADH genes will yield further insights into alcohol metabolism in humans.

The alcohol dehydrogenases of human have been divided into three distinct classes based on their physical and enzymatic properties. These three classes of ADHs show differences in tissue distribution and timing of expression. Although they are the principal enzymes involved in the metabolism of ethanol[1] and all metabolize ethanol to some degree, they also metabolize many other alcohols and so their physiological role is still uncertain. The enzymatic classes are distinguished by their Km for ethanol, sensitivity to inhi-

Robin W. Cotton and David Goldman are affiliated with the Section of Genetics, Laboratory of Clinical Studies, Division of Intramural Clinical and Biological Research, National Institute on Alcohol Abuse and Alcoholism, NIH Clinical Center, Bldg. 10, Rm. 3C218, Bethesda, MD 20892.

Reprint requests should be sent to David Goldman.

bition with 4-methyl pyrazole, and isoelectric point. All have a monomeric molecular weight of about 40,000, have an acetylated N-terminal, contain two zinc atoms and require NAD(H) for activity.[2]

ENZYMOLOGY

The enzymology of the class I alcohol dehydrogenases has been extensively studied. There are three class I genes, ADH 1, 2 and 3, coding for three protein subunits, α, β and γ. The holoenzymes are homo or hetero-dimers and the six combinations of monomeric subunits differ in their activity with various substrates.[3-5] The class I enzymes have isoelectric points ranging from 9-11, have a high affinity for ethanol and are inhibited by 4-methyl pyrazole.[6] The sequence of all three subunits has been determined by amino acid sequencing of β and γ and by DNA sequencing of cloned cDNAs of all three subunits.[7-12] The extent of homology in the coding sequences of the three subunits is 95.6% between β and γ, 95.1% between α and β and 94.0% between α and γ.[12]

Variants in primary amino acid structure have been discovered for both the β and γ class I ADH subunits. The γ variant ($\gamma2$) has a methionine instead of valine at position 276 but the isozymes $\gamma1 \gamma1$ and $\gamma2 \gamma2$ have similar enzymatic activities.[5] In contrast, the variant $\beta2 \beta2$, which has a histidine instead of an arginine at position 47, has a lower pH optimum and ins 80 fold increased in enzyme activity (at the lower pH) as compared to the $\beta1 \beta1$ isozyme. $\beta1\beta2$ heterodimers also show atypical pH profiles and are more active than $\beta1$ homodimers.[4,13,14] These atypical enzymes are found in approximately 85% of Orientals and probably contribute to the flushing response commonly seen in Orientals by producing acetaldehyde more rapidly.[15] An inactive genetic variant of mitochondrial aldehyde dehydrogenase (ALDH 1) is present in approximately 50% of Orientals.

These two functional genetic variants affecting sequential steps in the pathway for ethanol metabolism can interact synergistically to produce high acetaldehyde levels and a flushing response following ethanol ingestion. Epidemiologic studies have now provided evidence for a protective role against alcoholism for the functional variant of ALDH 1. Only 4% of Japanese alcoholics but 42% of a Japanese population sample were deficient for ALDH 1 and only 10% of Taiwanese alcoholics as compared to 35% of a control population were deficient.[16]

Class II ADH(ADH 4) is found primarily in liver and stomach and Class III ADH(ADH 5) is constitutively expressed in many tissues and is the only ADH in brain.[17-19] In their functional enzymatic properties, the class II and III ADHs differ from the class I enzymes in a number of major ways. The class II enzyme has a higher Km for ethanol (0.5-4.0 mM for class I and about 120 mM for class II) while ethanol is an extremely poor substrate for class III. These enzyme differences are also reflected in their affinity for other substrates, the extent of their inhibition by 4-methyl pyrazole, their pH optimum and the isoelectric points of the subunit, with the class III enzyme differing the most in these functional parameters.[18-20] Class II ADH has recently been cloned and both a peptide and DNA sequence determined. The DNA sequence shows 60-65% homology with the three Class I ADHs.[21]

Developmental and tissue-specific differences in the expression of the ADHs could be important for understanding ethanol's intoxicating and toxic effects, especially to the fetus. The class I ADH genes show both developmental and tissue specificity in their expression. Among the class I genes, only the α ADH 1 is expressed in early fetal liver, expression of the ADH 2 begins during the second trimester and expression of the ADH 3 begins shortly after birth. In adult tissue, all three class I ADH isozymes are found in liver along with the class II and class III enzymes. In stomach, intestine and kidney, mainly ADH 3 is expressed and only ADH 2 is expressed in lung.[17] These changes in subunit expression would result in differences in the activity of the available holoenzyme, but what the developmental significance of these differences might be is not known.

MOLECULAR BIOLOGY

cDNA clones coding for the α, β and γ subunits have been sequenced confirming the high degree of homology between the three genes and the differences at the DNA level between the polymorphic subunits of β and γ.[7-12] In addition, Duester et al. have isolated class I ADH genomic clones covering 33 kb around the α gene, 23 kb around the β gene and 25 kb around the γ gene. Using these clones they demonstrated that the number and sizes of Eco RI fragments seen in a genomic digest can be accounted for in the set of genomic clones suggesting that there are no class I ADH pseudogenes. Their study of a single clone containing the entire β ADH gene revealed that the β gene covers 15 kb and contains 9 exons and 8 introns.[11]

cDNA clones coding for the β polypeptide isolated by Duester et al., by Ikuta et al., and also by Heden et al. were found to have four polyadenylation signals.[9,10,22] Different size classes of mRNA hybridizing to class I ADH probes have been reported as have changes in the size classes of mRNA found in the fetus, infant and adult.[23] Also, when gene specific probes are used, the size classes of mRNA coding for each of the three subunits are not the same. At least some of the variation in the size of the β mRNA results from the use of different polyadenylation signals.[24] Understanding how the size differences in class I ADH mRNAs relate to differences in gene expression awaits further study.

CHROMOSOMAL MAPPING

The alcohol dehydrogenases constitute a multigene family. The class I ADH genes have been mapped to human chromosome 4 by hybridization of a cDNA probe for the ADH 2 gene to a CHO-human hybrid cell line containing only human chromosome 4.[25] More precise localization of the three Class I ADH genes to chromosome 4q21-4q24 was accomplished using a panel of human-rodent hybrid cell lines. This data also established that all three class I genes are in this region since the Eco RI fragments from all three genes could be accounted for.[26] Class III ADH has also been mapped to the q21-q24 region of chromosome 4.[27] The map position of the class II gene has not yet been established. Cloned class I ADH probes developed by Smith et al. recognize DNA restriction fragment polymorphisms (RFLPs) specific for each of the three class I genes.[28] These probes along with the appropriate restriction enzyme, sizes of the polymorphic fragments and approximate gene frequencies are shown in Table 1. Using the RFLPs recognized by pADH 36, Murray et al. have established that ADH 3 lies 10-15 cM distal to the DNA probe GIFN and 5 cM proximal to EGF (epidermal growth factor).[29] Thus, the map position for a class I ADH gene complex is established in relation to two flanking markers on human chromosome 4.

Definitive evidence that the three class I ADH genes on chromosome 4 exist as a cluster came from segregation analysis of restriction fragment polymorphisms (RFLPs) in a large family as well as physical mapping using pulsed field gel electrophoresis (PFGE) to identify large DNA fragments containing all three class I ADH genes.[20] In the transmission analysis for genetic linkage, DNA RFLPs recognized by pADH 36 (ADH 2), pADH 73 (ADH 3) and pADH 74 (ADH 3) were informative and were followed in Mormon pedigree K-1331. A recombination event between ADH 2 and ADH 3 was observed in one individual giving a maximum lod score of

TABLE 1

CLASS 1 ADH PROBES AND RFLPS*

GENE	PROBE RECOGNIZING POLYMORPHIC RFLP	RESTRICTION ENZYME	FRAGMENT SIZE IN KB†	RFLP FREQUENCY
ADH 1	pADH 53	Msp 1	10.0 6.8	ND§ ND
ADH 2	pADH 36	Rsa 1	1.0 0.5	0.60 (SE=0.11)¶ 0.40 (SE=0.11)
ADH 3	pADH 53	Msp 1	12.5 10.0	0.75 (SE=0.097) 0.25 (SE=0.097)
ADH 3	pADH 73	Msp 1	12.5 10.0	0.75 (SD=0.097) 0.25 (SD=0.097)
ADH 3	pADH74	Xba 1	4.4 3.3	0.75 (SD=0.097) 0.25 (SD=0.097)

* see reference 28
† KB=kilobase pairs
§ ND=not done
¶ SE=standard error

1.2 (odds of linkage 16/1) and indicating linkage between the β and γ genes.[20]

PFGE, which permits the electrophoretic resolution of DNA fragments from 10 kb to over 1000 kb in size,[31,32] was then used to more precisely establish the distance covered by the three class I genes. For PFGE DNA samples are prepared in agarose blocks in order to eliminate shearing of the molecules which occurs during routine isolation of DNA.[33] Samples in agarose were digested with a number of restriction enzymes (Not 1, Mlu 1, Sfi 1 and Sal 1 which cut infrequently and therefore produce large fragments) and then loaded directly into sample wells of the gel. DNA from the pulse field gels was transferred to nitrocellulose by the method of Southern[34] and hybridized to either pADH 36, pADH 53 or pADH 74 under conditions which (for all probes) allows cross hybridization of the probe to all three class I genes. The sizes of the hybridizing bands produced with the enzymes listed above are shown in Table 2. Since both Not 1 and Mlu 1 produce only a single band, this band must contain all three class I genes. Both Sal I and Sfi I produce three class I ADH hybridizing bands, indicating that each band generated by these enzymes probably contains a single class I gene. The sum of the sizes of the three bands is 830 kb and 1000 kb for the Sfi I and Sal I digests respectively, establishing that the class I ADH gene complex has a maximum size of 850 kb. Duester et al. have reported that the β gene is 15 kb in length.[11] Assuming that the α and γ genes are of approximately the same size, the minimum size of the gene complex can be estimated to be equal to 270 kb (the

TABLE 2

SIZES OF CLASS I HYBRIDIZING BANDS ON PFGE*

ENZYME	BAND SIZE IN KB†
Not 1	1000
Mlu 1	1000
Sal 1	400, 260, 170
Sfi 1	380, 350, 270

* see reference 30
† KB= kilobase pairs

smallest fragment in the SfiI digest) plus 30 kb (two times the size of the β gene). This estimation of the minimum size of the gene complex assumes that the smallest Sfi I fragment contains the smallest Sal I fragment and that both these fragments contain whichever class I gene is in the middle of the gene complex.[30]

EVOLUTION

The existence of a multigene family is a reflection of the evolutionary history of the gene family. Members of multigene families may be dispersed on different chromosomes (for example: α, cardiac and β actin on chromosomes 1, 15 and 7 respectively) or may be arranged close together as gene clusters (for example: the α globin cluster on chromosome 16pter-p12, the β globin cluster on chromosome 11p15.5).[34] In the formation of multigene families the initial gene duplication can result from a variety of events including homologous recombination between repeated sequences, insertion of DNA sequences formed from RNA intermediates or gene amplification resulting from several initiation events at a single origin of replication.[36] However the initial gene duplication occurs, subsequent recombination events such as gene conversion or unequal crossing over can increase or decrease the number of genes in the gene family, the extent of their homogeneity, and the types of genetic variants which will be observed at a locus.[36] For example, unequal crossing over at the α globin complex produces α thalassemias in which the number of functional α globin genes available is smaller than the normal complement due to abnormal crossing over between highly homologous sequences within the complex.[37]

Information from amino acid composition, enzymatic properties and amino acid and DNA sequence data can be examined for clues to the evolution of the ADH gene family. Like human, mouse has three distinct classes of ADH isozymes which exist as a gene complex on mouse chromosome 3.[38] The enzymatic properties of the three classes of mouse ADH are similar to the properties of the three ADH classes in humans although each mouse isozyme seems to be coded by a single gene.[39] Ikuta et al. have calculated a consensus DNA sequence from the three human class I coding sequences and compared the resulting amino acid sequence consensus to each human class I amino acid sequence and also to the amino acid sequence of the mouse class I like subunit (ADH-A) and the horse ADH-E. This comparison along with data presented by Edenberg et al. argue that mouse ADH-A, horse ADH-E and human ADH 2 had a common ancestral gene.[12,40]

Jörnvall et al. present an evolutionary scheme in which duplications of an ancestral ADH gene resulted in the three classes of ADH isozymes. Subsequent independent duplication events of the class I ancestor gene gave rise to the horse ADH-E and ADH-S genes and the three Human class I genes.[41] Ikuta et al. suggest that one duplication produced an α and a β-γ-like subunit followed later by a division of β and γ.[12] Hempel et al. also suggest that the three human class I ADH subunits have arisen from two separate but recent gene duplications.[42] Enzymes which have enzymatic characteristics similar to the human class I isozymes have been isolated from squirrel monkey (*Saimiri sciureus*) and rhesus monkey (*Macaca mulatta*).[43,44] Hybridization of the pADH 53 α subunit probe[28] to a Southern blot of Msp I digested DNA from human, orangutan, siamang and gorilla suggests that there are multiple class I ADH like sequences in all of these primate species. In this experiment, hybridization was done at high stringency to allow hybridization only to closely homologous sequences. As seen in Figure 1, the hybridization pattern in the primate samples is simple, with a maximum of six bands seen in the orangutan sample, four in siamang, three in gibbon and two in gorilla indicating that there are several closely related ADH sequences in these species. This data would suggest that the gene duplications leading to multiple class I genes in human occurred prior to divergence of the primates.

In summary, study of the ADH genes at the protein and DNA levels has led to insights in their genetic functional variants, timing and tissue specificity of expression and evolutionary origins. The knowledge that class I ADH genes are organized as complex on chromosome 4 may lead to additional understanding of the regulation of these genes and the functional significance of the changes in expression of the three subunits during development and the differences in the subunits expressed in different tissues.

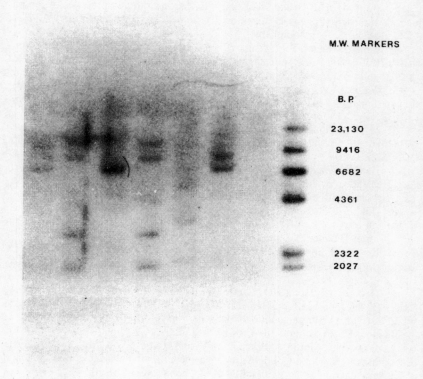

FIGURE 1. Autoradiogram of a southern blot hybridization showing the fragments recognized by class I probe pADH 53. Genomic DNA from the primates indicated across the top of the figure was digested with Msp I, separated by electrophoris on a 0.8% agarose gel, blotted onto nitrocellulose and hybridized at high stringency to [^{32}P] labeled pADH 53. [^{32}P] end labeled Hind III cut lambda DNA, seen in the far right, lane was used a molecular weight standard.

REFERENCES

1. Rognstad R, Grunnet N. Enzymatic pathways of ethanol metabolism. In: Majchrowicz E, ed. Biochemistry and Pharmacology of Ethanol. New York: Plenum Press. 1979; 1:65-85.

2. Strydom DJ, Vallee BL. Characterization of human alcohol dehydrogenase isozymes by high performance liquid chromatographic peptide mapping. Anal. Biochem. 1982; 123:422-429.

3. Smith M, Hopkinson DA, Harris H. Studies on the properties of the human alcohol dehydrogenase isozymes determined by the different loci ADH 1, ADH 2, ADH 3. Ann Hum Genet. 1973; 37:49-67.

4. Yin S-J, Bosron WF, Magnes LJ, Li T-K. Human liver alcohol dehydrogenase: Purification and kinetic characterization of the $\beta2 \beta2$, $\beta2 \beta1$, $\alpha \beta2$, and $\beta2 \gamma1$ "Oriental" isozymes. Biochem. 1984; 23:5847-5853.

5. Wagner FW, Burger AR, Vallee BL. Kinetic properties of human liver alcohol dehydrogenase: Oxidation of alcohols by class I isozymes. Biochemistry. 1983; 22:1857-1863.

6. Li TK, Magnes LJ. Identification of a distinctive molecular form of alcohol dehydrogenase in livers with high activity. Biochem Biophsy Res Commun. 1975; 63:202-208.

7. Hempel J, Bühler R, Kaiser R, Holmquist B, DE Zalenski C, Von Wartburg JP, Vallee B, Jörnvall H. Human liver alcohol dehydrogenase 1. The primary structure of the $\beta1 \beta1$ isozyme. Eur J Biochem. 1984; 145:437-445.

8. Bühler R, Hempel J, Kaiser R, DE Zalenski C, Von Wartburg JP, Jörnvall H. Human liver alcohol dehydrogenase 2. The primary structure of the $\gamma1$ protein chain. Eur J. Biochem. 1985; 145:447-453.

9. Ikuta T, Fujiyoshi T, Kurachi K, and Yoshida A. Molecular cloning of a full-length cDNA for human alcohol dehydrogenase. Proc Natl Acad Sci USA. 1985; 82:2703-2707.

10. Heden L-O, Höög J-O, Larsson K, Lake M. Lagerholm E, Holmgren A, Vallee BL, Jörnvall H, von Bahr-Lindström H. cDNA clones coding for the β-subunit of human liver alcohol dehydrogenase have differently sized 3'-non-coding regions. FEBS Letters. 1986; 194:327-332.

11. Duester G, Smith M, Bilanchone V, and Hatfield WG. Molecular analysis of the human class I alcohol dehydrogenase gene family and nucleotide sequence of the gene encoding the β subunit. J Biol Chem. 1986; 261:2027-2033.

12. Ikuta T, Szeto S, and Yoshida A. Three human alcohol dehydrogenase subunits: cDNA structure and molecular and evolutionary divergence. Proc Natl Acad Sci USA. 1986; 83:634-638.

13. Yoshida A, Impraim CC, Huang I-Y. Enzymatic and structural differences between usual and atypical human liver alcohol dehydrogenase. J Boil. Chem. 1981; 23:12430-12436.

14. Bühler R, Hempel J., von Wartburg J-P, Jörnvall H. Atypical human liver alcohol dehydrogenase: the $\beta2$-Bern subunit has an amino acid exchange that is identical to the one in the $\beta2$-Oriental chain. FEBS Letters. 1984; 173:360-366.

15. Stamatoyannopoulos G, Chen S-H, Fukui M. Liver alcohol dehydrogenase in Japanese: High population frequency of atypical form and its possible role in alcohol sensitivity. Am J Hum Genet. 1975; 27:789-796.

16. Ohmori T, Koyama T, Chen C-C, Yeh EK, Reyes BV, Yamashita I. The role of aldehyde dehydrogenase enzyme variance in alcohol sensitivity, drinking habits formation and the development of alcoholism in Japan, Taiwan and the Philippines. Prog Neuro-psychopharmacol Biol Psychiatry. 1986; 10:229-235.

17. Smith M. Hopkinson DA, Harris H. Developmental changes and polymorphism in human alcohol dehydrogenase. Ann Hum Genet. 1971; 34:251-271.

18. Beisswenger TB, Holmquist B, Vallee BL. chi- ADH is the sole alcohol dehydrogenase isozyme of mammalian brains: Implications and inferences. Proc Natl Acad Sci USA. 1985; 82:8369-8373.

19. Ditlow CC, Holmquist B, Morelock MM, Vallee BL. Physical and enzymatic properties of a class II alcohol dehydrogenase isozyme of human liver: pi-ADH. Biochemistry. 1984; 23:6363-6368.

20. Wagner FW, Parés X, Holmquist B, Vallee BL. Physical and enzymatic-properties of a class II isozyme of human liver alcohol dehydrogenase: chi-ADH. Biochemistry. 1984; 23:2193-2199.

21. Höög J-O, von Bahr-Lindström H, Hedén L-O, Holmquist B, Larsson K, Hempel J, Vallee BL, Jörnvall H. Structure of the class II enzyme of human liver alcohol dehydrogenase: Combined cDNA and protein sequence determination of the pi subunit. Biochemistry. 1987; 26:1926-1932.

22. Duester G, Hatfield WG, Bühler R, Hempel J, Jörnvall H, and Smith M. Molecular cloning and characterization of a cDNA for the β subunit of human alcohol dehydrogenase. Proc Natl Acad Sci USA. 1984; 81:4055-4059.

23. Bilanchone V, Duester G, Edwards Y, Smith M. Multiple mRNAs for human alcohol dehydrogenase (ADH): developmental and tissue specific differences. Nuc Acids Res. 1986; 14:3911-3926.

24. Ikuta T, Yoshida A. mRNA for the three human alcohol dehydrogenase subunits: size heterogeneity and developmental changes. Biochem Biophys Res Comm. 1986; 140:1020-1027.

25. Duester G. Hatfield WG, and Smith M. Molecular genetic analysis of human alcohol dehydrogenase. Alcohol. 1985; 2:53-56.

26. Smith M. Duester G. Carlock L, Wasmuth J. Assignment of ADH1, ADH2 and ADH3 genes (class I ADH) to human chromosome 4q21-4q25, through use of DNA probes. Human Gene Mapping 8. Cytogenet Cell Genet. 1985; 40:748.

27. Carlock L. Hiroshige S, Wasmuth J, and Smith M. Assignment of the ADH 5 gene coding for class II ADH to human chromosome 4:4q21-4q25. Human Gene Mapping 8. Cytogenet Cell Genet. 1985; 40:598.

28. Murray J, personal communication.

29. Smith M. Genetics of Human ADH and ALDH. Adv in Hum Genet. 1985; 15:259-290.

30. Cotton RW, Goldman D. A class I alcohol dehydrogenase gene complex on human chromosome 4. 1987 manuscript submitted.

31. Lawrance SK, Srivastava R, Rigas B, Chorney MJ, Gillespie GA, Smith CL, Cantor CR, Collins FS, and Weissman SM. Molecular approaches to the characterization of megabase regions of DNA: Applications to the human major histocompatibility complex. Cold Spring Harbor Symp Quant Biol. 1986; 51:123-130.

32. Hardy DA, Bell JI, Long EO, Lindsten T, and McDevitt HO. Mapping of the class II region of the human major histocompatibility complex by pulsed-field gel electrophoresis. Nature. 1986; 323:453-455.

33. Smith CL. Methods in Enzymology; in press.

34. Southern EM. Detection of specific sequences among DNA fragments separated by gel electrophoresis. J Mol Biol. 1975; 98:503-517.

35. de la Chapelle A. Human Gene Mapping 8: Eighth international workshop on human gene mapping. Cytogenet Cell Genet. 1985; 40:128-155.

36. Maeda N, Smithies O. The evolution of multigene families: Human haptoglobin genes. Ann Rev Genet. 1986; 20:81-108.

37. Kan YW. Molecular pathology of α-thalassemia. Ann NY Acad Sci. 1985; 445:28-35.

38. Holmes RS, Duley JA, Burnell JN. The alcohol dehydrogenase gene complex on chromosome 3 of the mouse. Isozymes: Current Topics in Biol and Med Res. 1983; 8:155-174.

39. Algar EM, Seeley T-L, Holmes RS. Purification and molecular properties of mouse alcohol dehydrogenase isozymes. Eur J Biochem. 1983; 137:139-147.

40. Edenberg HJ, Zhang K, Fong K. Bosron WF, Li T-K. Cloning and sequencing of cDNA encoding the complete mouse liver alcohol dehydrogenase. Proc Natl Acad Sci USA. 1985; 82:2262-2266.

41. Jörnvall H, Höög JO, von Bahr-Lindström H, and Vallee BL. Mammalian alcohol dehydrogenases of separate classes: Intermediates between different enzymes and intraclass isozymes. Proc Natl Acad Sci USA. 1987; 84:2580-2584.

42. Hempel J, Holmquist B, Fleetwood L, Kaiser R, Barros-Söderling J, Bühler R, Vallee BL, Jörnvall H. Structural relationships among class I isozymes of human liver alcohol dehydrogenase. Biochemistry. 1985; 24:5303-5307.

43. Dafeldecker WP, Parés X, Vallee, BL, Bosron WF, Li TK. Simian liver alcohol dehydrogenase: Isolation and characterization of isozymes from *Saimiri sciureus*. Biochemistry. 1981; 20:856-861.

44. Dafeldecker WP, Meadow PE, Parés X, Vallee BL. Simian liver alcohol dehydrogenase: Isolation and characterization of isozymes from *Macaca mulatta*. Biochemistry. 1981; 20:6729-6734.

Polyunsaturated Fatty Acids
and Ethanol

Norman Salem, Jr., PhD
John W. Karanian, PhD

SUMMARY. Ethanol exposure leads to a loss in membrane polyunsaturated fatty acids (PUFA). It is proposed that polyunsaturated species of phospholipids are not randomly distributed, but are concentrated in the cytosolic leaflets of the plasma membrane and are preferentially associated with membrane proteins. These lipids affect the physical state of environments surrounding membrane proteins and thereby serve to regulate many cellular functions. Disruption of these environments may occur even when a small percentage of total polyunsaturates is lost due to ethanol exposure. One possible mechanism of ethanol-induced polyunsaturate loss may be activation of a phospholipase A_2 enzyme which is selective for these species of phospholipids. Fatty acids released would stimulate the production of prostaglandins and/or leukotrienes. Similarly, the released docosahexaenoate can be metabolized by rat brain to leukotriene-like compounds which are biologically active in smooth muscle systems. This metabolism is stimulated by ethanol in human platelets, *in vitro*.

INTRODUCTION

Several investigators have demonstrated that ethanol exposure can lead to changes in polyunsaturated lipid content in various biological tissues.[1] It is therefore important to consider what the biological implications of altered polyunsaturate levels and metabolism might be. It is possible that losses of these lipids may lead to cell

Norman Salem, Jr. and John W. Karanian are affiliated with the Section of Analytical Chemistry, Laboratory of Clinical Studies, Division of Intramural Clinical and Biological Research, National Institute on Alcohol Abuse and Alcoholism, NIH Clinical Center, Bldg. 10, Rm. 3C-218, Bethesda, MD 20892.

Reprint requests should be sent to Norman Salem, Jr.

death and ultimately to organ pathology such as is associated with alcoholic dementia or cirrhosis of the liver. Losses of brain 22:6w3 are known to be associated with several neurological disorders.[2] In addition, two other possible ramifications of altered polyunsaturated fatty acid metabolism must be considered. These are the alteration of the physical properties of cell membranes and altered formation of potent, bioactive fatty acid metabolites such as prostaglandins or leukotrienes. This report will focus upon both of these issues with an emphasis upon the development of new approaches and techniques for the elucidation of ethanol action.

Littleton[3] and coworkers have observed a somewhat selective decrease in docosahexaenoic acid (22:6w3) in both mouse heart and brain after ethanol inhalation for two hours (fatty acids are denoted using the format "X:YwZ," where 'X' is the number of carbons in the chain, 'Y' is the number of double bonds and 'Z' is the number of carbons from the methyl end to the first double bond). However, a decrease in brain (P_2 fraction) arachidonate (20:4w6) was also observed after 10 days of ethanol exposure.[3] Rat liver extracts generally show a decrease in arachidonate and a compensatory increase in linoleate (18:2w6) after ethanol exposure.[1] Aloia et al.[4] demonstrated losses of 20:4w6, 22:6w3 and 22:3w6 in various phospholipid classes of rat cortex microsomes after 35 days of an ethanol-supplemented liquid diet. Cursted[5] also found a 20:4w6 decline in rat liver phospholipids after ethanol feeding but observed an increase in 22:6w3. Sun and Sun[6] found that ethanol exposure led to increased levels of 22:4 and 22:6w3 in guinea pig synaptosomal phosphatidylethanolamines. However, Harris et al.[7] reported a highly selective decrease in 22:6w3 in mouse brain after 7 days of an ethanol-containing liquid diet. There was a selective decline of 22:6w3 in phosphatidylserines only. They found no significant changes in the levels of any phospholipid class. Losses of polyunsaturates have also been observed in alcoholic patients during withdrawal. For example, Alling et al.[8] reported a decline in both 20:4w6 and 22:6w3 in erythrocyte phospholipids during the first two weeks after withdrawal onset. In another study, arachidonate and other polyunsaturates were significantly reduced in erythrocyte and plasma phospholipids in alcoholics but fatty acid supplements partially reversed these w-6 fatty acid losses.[9] In contrast, LaDroitte et al.[10] reported no significant decreases in polyunsaturates in erythrocyte membrane phospholipids from alcoholics. Although there is disagreement concerning both the amount and, in some cases, the direction of changes in fatty acyl content of blood cells and organs after ethanol exposure, it is difficult to directly compare these studies. In order to rigorously compare such results, many variables need to be controlled including the mode of ethanol delivery, the level and duration of exposure, the diet composition and the particular tissue, species and lipid class under investigation. Still, it would appear that the weight of evidence would favor the proposition that ethanol exposure leads to a decline in the polyunsaturated fatty acyl content of cell membranes.

METHODS

Total lipids were extracted using the procedure of Bligh and Dyer.[11] Phospholipid classes were separated using a two dimensional TLC system modified from that of Rouser.[12] Fatty acid methyl esters were formed by reaction with BF_3 in methanol.[13] Erythrocytes were labelled with trinitrobenzenesulfonate (TNBS) and the phosphatidylethanolamine derivatives formed were separated by HPLC as previously described.[14] Exposure of rats to ethanol was performed using the inhalation method of Karanian et al.[15] One ml of platelets (10^8 cells/ml) was incubated for 20 min at 37°.C with 0.25 uC of 1-^{14}C-docosahexaenoic acid (22:6w3) and 35 ug of unlabelled 22:6w3 in a 0.2M tris-HCl, pH 7.5 buffer containing 10 mM EDTA.[16] Metabolite extraction and HPLC separation were performed as described by Shingu[16,17] and mass spectral analysis as described by Yergey et al.[18]

RESULTS AND DISCUSSION

Membrane Physical Properties

The study of the modification of the physical state of cell membranes by alcohols was pioneered by Goldstein and coworkers.[19-21] Alcohols added to membranes *in vitro* have a disordering effect on

membrane constituents which is often referred to as "fluidization."[19] Cell membranes appear to adapt to chronic ethanol exposure by becoming more rigid.[20] They also become less responsive to
the disordering action of ethanol and this has been referred to as the
"membrane tolerance" phenomenon.[6,20-24] Similar changes in erythrocyte membranes from alcoholics have been observed both with
respect to membrane fluidity and tolerance.[25] It is known that polyunsaturated phospholipids can mediate changes in the physical state
of membranes.[26] Membrane fluidity is directly related to the level of
polyunsaturated fatty acids in component phospholipids.[27] Phospholipid extracts or individual phospholipid classes purified from ethanol-fed rats are capable of conferring membrane tolerance to liposomal membranes.[22,24] Therefore, changes in the levels or possibly the
topographic localization or molecular association of polyunsaturated phospholipids associated with ethanol exposure may be an
important aspect of its drug action.

Fatty Acid and Phospholipid Species Composition

Male, Sprague-Dawley rats were exposed to ethanol vapor for 1-
14 days in specially designed inhalation chambers.[15] Total lipid extracts were made of various organs and tissues, and fatty acid profiles were compiled after transmethylation. Various phospholipid
classes had quite distinct fatty acid profiles. Losses of arachidonate
were apparent in the liver, aorta, erythrocyte and platelet but were
smaller in the heart and brain. The most striking alterations were
found in the fatty acid content of the liver, and therefore individual
phospholipids were investigated. Losses of polyunsaturates were
most marked in the acidic phospholipids, phosphatidylserine (PS)
and phosphatidylinositol (PI), but phosphatidylethanolamine (PE)
was little affected. For example, the arachidonate (20:4w6) decline
after 14 days of ethanol inhalation in PS, PI, PC and PE was 64, 53,
49 and 16%, and the docosahexaenoate decline was 30, 38, 28 and
3%, respectively. The blood ethanol concentration was about 200
mg% in these animals. It is important to note that the liver total lipid
extract showed only a 20% decline in 20:4w6 and no decline in
22:6w3. It should be apparent from these data that ethanol-induced
alterations in PUFA can be selective for particular lipid classes or

particular molecular species and that such changes can be missed if analyses are carried out solely on total lipid extracts.

We have previously reported on ethanol-induced alterations in the distributions of liver microsomal PI molecular species in samples that are capable of conferring resistance to the disordering effects of ethanol (membrane tolerance). There was a drop in the three arachidonyl-PI species that were determined and a concomitant increase in other w-6 PI species in the ethanol exposed membranes.[14] However, fatty acid analysis shows only a 10% change in the total arachidonate level. It is somewhat difficult to see how this minor change in fatty acid distribution could cause such a profoundly different response of the cell or liposomal membranes when challenged with ethanol. Previous work has demonstrated a direct link between the degree of unsaturation of phospholipids and membrane fluidity. For example, the degree of disorder of a cholestane probe in PS liposomes varied directly with the 22:6w3 content.[27] Therefore, loss in membrane polyunsaturates might explain a baseline change in membrane fluidity such as has been observed after chronic ethanol exposure.[20] Although polyunsaturates are clearly involved in the maintenance of the proper physical state of the membrane, it is still unclear by what mechanism their loss may mediate a resistance to the disordering effects of ethanol. Some type of signal amplification is needed in order for these compositional changes to exert such effects.

There are several possibilities for ways in which fatty acyl compositional changes induced by ethanol exposure can have a marked impact on the cell membrane state. It is possible that new phospholipid species are formed which have very different physical properties than species that they replace. For example, Van Deenen et al.[28] and Kuypers et al.[29] have found that replacing erythrocyte PC with diunsaturated PC led to a progressive increase in osmotic fragility, shape changes, ionic permeability and hemolysis. A second possibility involves the specialization of membrane microenvironments so as to concentrate particular phospholipid species together and in this way amplify their physical properties.[2] A third possibility involves the metabolism of PUFA to potent, biologically active compounds. These latter two possibilities will be the subject of the remainder of this paper.

Membrane Microenvironments

It has long been known that there is a nonrandom distribution of various lipid classes on the two leaflets of the plasma membrane.[30,31] Phosphatidylethanolamine (PE) is asymmetrically localized in the plasma membrane of many cells with about one-third on the cell surface.[30] The reasons for this element of membrane structure and the means by which it is maintained, if any, are largely unknown. One possible contributory factor might be the very different fatty acyl side chains present in the PE. The hypothesis that there was asymmetry with respect to differences in acyl content within one phospholipid class in cell membranes was tested and verified in human lymphocytes and several cultured cell lines[32] and in the erythrocyte as well.[14] It was generally observed that polyunsaturated species of PE were preferentially localized on the cytoplasmic leaflet of plasma membranes whereas monoenoic species were more often found on the cell surface. This phenomenon may be termed a phospholipid molecular species asymmetry and is believed to be a common feature of cell membranes.[2] Such asymmetry was also recently observed in trout intestinal brush border membranes.[33]

A second type of specialization that has been observed in plasma membranes involves the molecular associations of phospholipids with membrane proteins. Aminophospholipids can be covalently crosslinked to protein amino groups using difluorodinitrobenzene.[34] This technique can be modified so that fatty acid composition of the phospholipids thus crosslinked to proteins can be analyzed.[35] In this way, it was found that the hexaenoic species of aminophospholipids were preferentially associated with proteins in neural membranes.[35] This phenomenon has also been observed in several cultured cell lines (N. Salem, unpublished).

Taken together, the findings that polyunsaturates are fluidizing and that they are preferentially localized on the plasma membrane interior and in domains surrounding membrane proteins have great biological significance. It has been proposed that polyunsaturated aminophospholipids such as 22:6-PS or 20:4-PE may exert a regulatory role for many cellular processes. This has been confirmed, for example, for PS and opiate receptor binding.[35,36] The fluidizing effect of 18:0, 22:6-PS[27] would be amplified when these lipid species are concentrated in a particular environment. For the PS species, in particular, it is also possible to modulate the fluidity of these environments by "freezing" them by means of an increased calcium concentration.[37] The polyunsaturates may thus serve to impart a greater dynamic range to the mobility of molecules which compose these membrane microenvironments. Consistent with this hypothesis is the observation that ESR probes which sample the membrane interior leaflet exhibit greater fluidity than cell surface probes.[38] Since, as previously discussed, ethanol exposure leads to a decline in polyunsaturated phospholipid levels, one of the important consequences may be the depletion of these microenvironments. A small change in membrane fluidity may result especially if a reporter molecule is used which partitions preferentially into bilayer regions of the membrane. This would reflect a much larger magnitude change in the areas where these lipids are concentrated. The possible disturbances of these protein-lipid interactions by acute ethanol exposure (due to its effects on hydrophobic binding) may be a factor in the fluidizing characteristics of ethanol observed for the membrane bilayer. One possibility is that exposure may lead to a greater amount of these polyunsaturated species present in those membrane bilayer areas where they may be more often sensed by fluorescent or ESR probe molecules; thus an increase in "membrane fluidity" would be observed. Actually, a redistribution of the fluidizing molecules in the membrane to form a more random configuration would be adopted in response to ethanol. During chronic exposure to ethanol, the destruction of this aspect of membrane specialization may help to explain why subsequent fluidization is not observed when ethanol is added *in vitro* (membrane tolerance). It could also explain how a 10 or 20% loss of polyunsaturated species might result in significant changes in both membrane function and physical properties.

One final aspect of this hypothesis involves the question of by what mechanism ethanol exposure is able to cause losses in polyunsaturates. Any of a number of processes whereby cells accumulate, biosynthesize, modify and catabolize fatty acids could be affected. An interesting possibility might be the activation of phospholipase

A_2. Indeed, an activating effect of ethanol on this enzyme has been observed.[39] This would be expected to preferentially release unsaturated fatty acids since the sn-2 position of phospholipids is attacked. Salem has shown that bee venom phospholipase A_2 releases polyunsaturates in preference to monoenes in neural membranes[40,2] and has proposed that this may be a feature of endogenous enzyme.[2] This characteristic has also been observed in two snake venom enzyme preparations.[41] Taken together, it would seem that ethanol may, at least potentially, be expected to activate a phospholipase which has a substrate preference for polyunsaturates and in this way cause a decline in their levels. Consistent with this hypothesis is the recent report that ethanol causes a rapid release of arachidonate (20:4w6) from mouse peritoneal macrophages.[42]

Oxygenated Metabolites

Finally, the last major possibility which will be discussed regarding mechanisms through which ethanol may exert powerful effects on cellular function through modification of lipid components is the modification of pathways involved in enzymatic oxygenation. It has long been known that unsaturated fatty acids like arachidonate (20:4w6) can be converted by cyclooxygenase or lipoxygenase enzymes into potent, bioactive compounds such as prostaglandins or leukotrienes. These so-called eicosanoids have important functions in many different organs and cell types.[43] Their importance in alcohol research was suggested in a report by Linnoila et al. that some cyclooxygenase inhibitors (e.g., indomethacin) could partially reverse the effects of alcohol on psychomotor skills in humans.[44] The antagonistic effect of indomethacin on behavioral responses to ethanol has been confirmed and related to brain prostaglandin levels.[45-47] Horrobin has hypothesized that acute ethanol stimulates the conversion of 20:3w6 to prostaglandin E_1 (PGE_1) but that chronic exposure leads to a decline in this fatty acid precursor due to desaturase inhibition and, consequently, a decline in its prostanoid metabolite.[48] Alcoholics may then increase their alcohol intake in order to maintain their PGE_1 levels. Anggard has proposed a similar hypothesis to account for ethanol effects on both one- and two-series prostaglandins.[49] Karanian and Salem have carefully studied the relationship of prostanoid production to both ethanol concentration and duration of exposure in isolated rat aortic strips and observed a stimulation in prosta-cyclin and thromboxane catabolites.[50,51] Chronic exposure (14 days) to ethanol vapors leads to a decline in prostanoid production and this was correlated with a decline in their precursor, arachidonic acid (20:4w6) in this tissue.[51] These prostanoids were abnormal in the urine of alcoholics during withdrawal.[52] High levels of ethanol lead to increases in lipoxygenase products as well.[53] Differences in both cyclooxygenase and lipoxygenase products have been ob-served in mice strains bred for their differing sensitivities to etha-nol.[54] These studies have suggested an important role for polyunsat-urates and their eicosanoid metabolites in mediating some of the biochemical abnormalities associated with alcohol intake. We have hypothesized that there is an analogous metabolic system operating on 22:6w3 in brain[2,16-18] and other tissues.[16,17] Previous work has indi-cated the presence of an enzymatic system in rat brain *in vitro* capa-ble of producing various oxygenated metabolites of exogenously added 22:6w3.[2,17,18] An accompanying paper in this volume has ex-tended this work to human platelets[16] in confirmation of the findings of Alvedano et al.[55] More importantly, it is shown that compounds with chromatographic behavior similar to the platelet 11- and 14-hydroxy-docosahexaenoate are produced both *in vitro* and *in vivo* by rat brain. This is the first report of 22:6w3 metabolism *in vivo* in a mammalian organism. It is herein reported that ethanol added to human platelets is capable of stimulating hydroxy-22:6w3 produc-tion (Table 1). A small (11-14%) but statistically significant stimu-lation can be observed in the upper part of the physiological range with respect to blood ethanol levels (i.e., 400-800mg%). This stim-ulation is of much greater magnitude (170%) when examined in rat platelets *in vitro* after the animals have been subjected to ethanol inhalation for seven days. These findings are consistent with the previously discussed decline in 22:6w3 in brain and other tissues after ethanol exposure. The metabolites formed are biologically ac-tive as they are capable of inducing smooth muscle contraction and of antagonizing the effects of other contractile agents.[16] The partial blockade of the contractile effect of the 22:6w3 metabolite by li-poxygenase but not cyclooxygenase inhibitors provides indirect evi-dence for modulation of leukotriene production by hydroxylated-22:6w3.[16]

Several aspects of the hypothesis presented above are summa-

Table 1. Stimulating effect of ethanol on hydroxy-docosahexeanoic acid production in human platelets in vitro.

	PICOMOLES/MIN/10^9 CELLS	%CHANGE
CONTROL	210 ± 10	—
ETHANOL (MG%)		
200	219 ± 12	+4
400	232 ± 11*	+11
800	239 ± 17*	+14
1600	265 ± 24**	+26
3200	289 ± 32**	+38

* Denotes significance at p<0.05 and ** p<0.01.

rized in a model (Figure 1). Schematically depicted is a hexaenoic species of PS on the plasma membrane interior and associated with a membrane protein. Ethanol exposure causes a decline in these polyunsaturated species which may, at least partially, be mediated by the stimulation of endogenous phospholipase A_2 which has a substrate selectivity for these species. Polyunsaturates released can then be metabolized to prostaglandins or leukotrienes. Docosahex-aenoic acid is also metabolized to leukotriene-like structures by brain and platelets and ethanol can stimulate such conversion, *in vitro*. Biological function is affected in two ways. The loss in poly-unsaturated phospholipids depletes an important lipid pool which is postulated to have a modulatory role in the function of membrane proteins. Secondly, fatty acids released from membranes may be metabolized to oxygenated compounds which are potent modulators of many cellular functions.

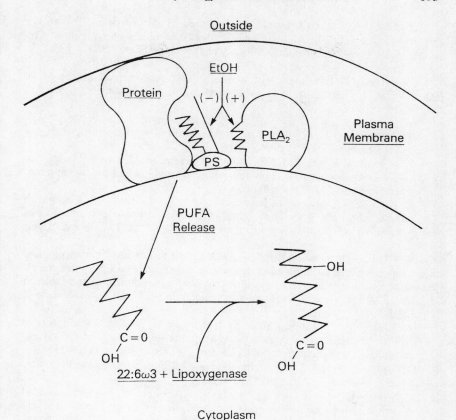

FIGURE 1. Schematic representation of the effects of ethanol on polyunsaturates in membranes.

REFERENCES

1. Reitz RC. The effects of ethanol ingestion on lipid metabolism. Prog Lipid Res. 1979; 18:87-115.

2. Salem Jr N, Kim H-Y, Yergey JA. Docosahexaenoic acid: membrane function and metabolism. In: Simopoulos AP, Kifer RR, Martin R, eds. Health effects of polyunsaturated fatty acids in seafoods. New York: Academic Press, 1986; 263-317.

3. Littleton JM, John GR, Grieve SJ. Alterations in phospholipid composition in ethanol tolerance and dependence. Alcoholism: Clin Exper Res. 1979; 3:50-6.

4. Aloia RC, Paxton J, Daviau JS, Van Geib O, Miekusch W, Truppe W, Meyer JA, Brauer FS. Effect of chronic alcohol consumption on rat brain microsome lipid composition, membrane fluidity and Na$^+$K$^+$ATPase activity. Life Sci. 1985; 36:1003-17.

5. Curstedt T. Biosynthesis of molecular species of hepatic glycerophosphatides during metabolism of [1,1-^{2}H]-ethanol in rats. Biochim Biophys Acta. 1982; 713:589-601.

6. Sun GY, Sun AY. Effect of chronic ethanol administration on phospholipid acyl groups of synaptic plasma membrane fraction isolated from guinea pig brain. Res Commun Chem Path Pharmacol. 1979; 24:405-8.

7. Harris BA, Baster DM, Mitchell MA, Hitzemann RJ. Physical properties and lipid composition of brain membranes from ethanol tolerant-dependent mice. Molecular Pharmacol. 1984; 25:401-9.

8. Alling C, Gustavsson L, Krisstensson-Aas A, Wallerstedt S. Changes in fatty acid composition of major glycerophospholipids in erythrocyte membranes from chronic alcoholics during withdrawal. Scand J Clin Lab Invest. 1984; 44:283-9.

9. Glen E, MacDonnell L, Glen I, MacKenzie J. Possible pharmacological approaches to the prevention and treatment of alcohol related CNS impairment: results of a double blind trial of essential fatty acids. In: Edwards G and Littleton J, eds. Pharmacological treatments for alcoholism. New York: Methuen, 1984:331-50.

10. LaDroitte P, Lamboeuf Y, de Saint Blanquat G, Bezaury J-P. Sensitivity of individual erythrocyte membrane phospholipid changes in fatty acid composition in chronic alcoholic patients. Alcoholism: Clin Exper Res. 1984; 9:135-7.

11. Bligh G, Dyer WJ. A rapid method of total lipid extraction and purification. Can J Biochem Physiol. 1959; 37:911-7.

12. Rouser G, Kritchevsky G, Yamamoto A. Column chromatographic and associated procedures for separation and determination of phosphatides and glycolipids. In: Marinetti GV, ed. Lipid chromatographic analysis, v.1. New York: Marcel Dekker, 1967; 1:99-162.

13. Morrison WR, Smith LM. Preparation of fatty acid methyl esters and dimethylacetals from lipids with boron floride-methanol. J Lipid Res. 1964; 5:600-8.

14. Salem Jr N, Yoffe A, Kim H-Y, Karanian JW, Taraschi TF. Effects of fish oils and alcohol on polyunsaturated lipids in membranes. In: Lands WEM, ed. Polyunsaturated fatty acids and eicosanoids. Champaign: Amer Oil Chemists Soc., 1987:185-91.

15. Karanian JW, Yergey J, Lister R, D'Souza N, Linnoila M, Salem Jr. N. Characterization of an automated apparatus for precise control of inhalation chamber ethanol vapor and blood ethanol concentrations. Alcoholism: Clin Exper Res. 1986; 10:443-7.

16. Shingu T, Karanian JW, Kim H-Y, Yergey JA, Salem Jr N. Discovery of novel brain lipoxygenase products formed from docosahexaenoic acid (22:6w3). Adv Alcohol Substance Abuse. 1988; 7(3/4):233-238.

17. Shingu T, Salem Jr N. Role of oxygen radical in peroxidation of docosahexaenoic acid by rat brain homogenate *in vitro*. In: Walden Jr TL, Hughes HN, eds. Prostaglandins and lipid metabolism in radiation injury. New York: Plenum Press, 1987 (in press).

18. Yergey J, Kim H-Y, Salem Jr N. High performance liquid chromatography-thermospray mass spectrometry of eicosanoids and novel oxygenated metabolites of docosahexaenoic acid. Anal Chem. 1986; 58:1344-8.

19. Chin JH, Goldstein DB. Effects of low concentrations of ethanol on the fluidity of spin-labeled erythrocyte and brain membranes. Mol Pharmacol. 1977; 13:435-41.

20. Lyon RC, Goldstein DB. Changes in synaptic membrane order associated with chronic ethanol treatment in mice. Mol Pharmacol. 1983; 23:86-91.

21. Chin JH, Goldstein DB. Drug tolerance in biomembranes: A spin label study of the effects of ethanol. Science. 1977; 196:684-5.

22. Taraschi TF, Ellingson JS, Rubin E. Membrane structural alterations caused by chronic ethanol consumption: the molecular basis of membrane tolerance. Annal New York Acad Sci. 1987; 492:171-80.

23. Taraschi TF, Ellingson JS, Wu A, Zimmerman R, Rubin E. Membrane tolerance to ethanol is rapidly lost after withdrawal: A model for studies of membrane adaptation. Proc Natl Acad Sci. 1986; 83:3669-73.

24. Taraschi TF, Ellingson JS, Wu A, Zimmerman R, Rubin E. Phosphatidylinositol from ethanol-fed rats confers membrane tolerance to ethanol. Proc Natl Acad Sci. 1986; 83:9398-402.

25. Beauge F, Stibler H, Borg S. Abnormal fluidity and surface carbohydrate content of the erythrocyte membrane in alcoholic patients. Alcohol: Clin Exper Res. 1985; 9:322-6.

26. Stubbs CD, Smith AD. The modification of mammalian membrane polyunsaturated fatty acid composition in relation to membrane fluidity and function. Biochim Biophys Acta. 1984; 779:89-137.

27. Salem Jr N, Serpentino P, Puskin JS, Abood LG. Preparation and spectroscopic characterization of molecular species of brain phosphatidylserines. Chem Phys Lipids. 1980; 27:289-304.

28. Van Deenen LLM, Kuypers FA, Op Den Kamp JAF, Roelofson B. Effects of altered phospholipid molecular species on erythrocyte membranes. Annal New York Acad Sci. 1987; 492:145-55.

29. Kuypers PA, Roelofsen B, Op Den Kamp JAF, Van Deenen LLM. The membrane of intact human erythrocytes tolerates only limited changes in the fatty acid composition of its phosphatidylcholine. Biochim Biophys Acta. 1984; 769:337-47.

30. Gordesky SE, Marinetti GV. The asymmetric arrangement of phospholipids in the human erythrocyte membrane. Biochem Biophys Res Commun. 1973; 50:1027-31.

31. Zwaal RFA, Roelofsen B, Comfurius P, Van Deenen LLM. Organization of phospholipids in human red cell membranes as detected by the action of various phospholipases. Biochim Biophys Acta. 1975; 406:83-96.

32. Bougnoux P, Salem Jr N, Lyons C, Hoffman T. Alteration in the membrane fatty acid composition of human lymphocytes and cultured transformed cells induced by interferon. Mol Immunol. 1985; 22:1107-13.

33. Pelletier X, Mersel M, Freysz L, Leray C. Topological distribution of aminophospholipid fatty acids in trout intestinal brush-border membrane. Biochem Biophys Acta. 1987; 902:223-8.

34. Gordesky SE, Marinetti GV, Segel GB. The interaction of 1-fluoro-2,4-dinitrobenzene with amino-phospholipids in membranes of intact erythrocytes, modified erythrocytes and erythrocyte ghosts. J Membrane Biol. 1973; 14:229-42.

35. Abood LG, Salem Jr N, MacNeil M, Bloom L, Abood ME. Enhancement of opiate binding by various molecular forms of phosphatidylserine and inhibition by other unsaturated lipids. Biochim Biophys Acta. 1977; 468:51-62.

36. Abood LG, Salem Jr N, MacNeil M, Butler M. Phospholipid changes in synaptic membranes by lipolytic enzymes and subsequent restoration of opiate binding with phosphatidylserine. Biochim Biophys Acta. 1978; 530:35-46.

37. Papahadjopoulos D, Poste G. Calcium-induced phase separation and fusion in phospholipid membranes. Biophysical J. 1975; 15:945-8.

38. Tanaka K, Ohnishi S. Heterogeneity in the fluidity of intact erythrocyte membrane and its homogenization upon hemolysis. Biochim Biophys Acta. 1976; 426:218-36.

39. Jain MH, Cordes EH. Phospholipases I. Effect of n-alkanols on the rate of enzymatic hydrolysis of egg phosphatidylcholine. J Membrane Biol. 1973; 144:101-18.

40. Salem Jr N. Preparation and spectroscopic characterization of molecular species of brain phosphatidylserine. PhD thesis, University of Rochester School of Medicine, 1978.

41. Butler M, Abood LG. Use of phospholipase A to compare phospholipid organization in synaptic membranes, myelin and liposomes. J Membrane Biol. 1982; 66:1-7.

42. Diez E, Balsinde J, Aracil M, Schuller A. Ethanol induces release of arachidonic acid but not synthesis of eicosanoids in mouse peritoneal macrophages. Biochim Biophys Acta. 1987; 921:82-9.

43. Wolfe L. Eicosanoids: prostaglandins, thromboxames, leukotrienes, and other derivatives of carbon-20 unsaturated fatty acids. J Neurochem. 1982; 38:1-14.

44. Linnoila M, Seppala T, Mattila MJ. Acute effect of antipyretic analgesics, alone or in combination with alcohol, on human psychomotor skills related to driving. Br J Clin Pharmac. 1974; 1:477-84.

45. George FR, Collins AC. Ethanol's behavioral effects may be partly due to increases in brain prostaglandin production. Alcoholism: Clin Exper Res. 1985; 9:143-6.

46. Collins AC, Gilliam DM, Miner LL. Indomethacin pretreatment blocks the effects of high concentrations of ethanol. Alcoholism: Clin Exper Res. 1985; 9:271-376.

47. George FR, Ritz MC, Elmer GI, Collins AC. Time course of ethanol's effects on brain prostaglandins in LS and SS mice. Life Sci. 1986; 39:1069-75.

48. Horrobin DF. A biochemical basis for alcoholism and alcohol-induced damage including the fetal alcohol syndrome and cirrhosis: interference with essential fatty acid and prostaglandin metabolism. Med Hypotheses. 1980; 6:929-42.

49. Anggard E. Ethanol, essential fatty acids and prostaglandins. Pharmacol Biochem Behavior. 1983; 18:401-7.

50. Karanian JW, Stojanov M. Salem Jr N. Effects of ethanol on prostacyclin and thromboxane A_2 synthesis in rat aortic rings *in vitro*. Prostaglandins Leukotrienes Med. 1985; 175-86.

51. Karanian JW, Salem Jr N. Interaction of alcohol and prostaglandins in the vascular system: Implications for cardiovascular disease. In: Gallo LL, ed. Cardiovascular Diseases. New York: Plenum Press, 1987:299-321.

52. Neiman J, Hillbom M, Benthin G, Anggard EE. Urinary excretion of 2,3-dinor, 6-keto prostaglandin F_1-alpha and platelet thromboxane formation during ethanol withdrawal in alcoholics. J Clin Pathol. 1987; 40:512-5.

53. Westcott JY, Murphy RC. Effects of alcohols on arachidonic acid metabolism in murine mastocytoma cells and human polymorphonuclear leukocytes. Biochim Biophys Acta. 1985; 833:262-71.

54. Fradin A, Henson PM, Murphy RC. The effect of ethanol on arachidonic acid metabolism in the murine peritoneal macrophage. Prostaglandins. 1987; 33:579-89.

55. Alvedano MI, Sprecher H. Synthesis of hydroxy fatty acids from 4,7,10,13,16,19-[1-^{14}C] docosahexaenoic acid by human platelets. J Biol Chem. 1983; 258:9339-43.

Induction of Rat Hepatic Microsomal Drug Metabolizing Enzymes by Pyrazole and 4-Substituted Pyrazoles

A. L. Hayes, BS
L. J. Marden, PhD
M. V. McGuire, BS
N. W. Cornell, PhD

SUMMARY. Pyrazole and 4-methylpyrazole are potent inhibitors of liver alcohol dehydrogenase and as such have been proposed as potential antidotes to alcohol poisoning. These drugs are also inducers of hepatic cytochrome P-450. We tested pyrazole and four 4-substituted pyrazoles for their potential as inducers of cytochrome P-450 and drug metabolism in mature male rats. Total cytochrome P-450 was significantly increased ($p < 0.05$) 1.3 fold by treatment with 4-methylpyrazole. P-nitrophenol hydroxylase (PNPH) activity (nmol/min/mg protein) was increased 1.9 fold following treatment with pyrazole and with 4-methylpyrazole. Treatment with 4-methylpyrazole also resulted in a 2.9 fold increase in ethoxyresorufin deethylase (EROD) activity. In addition, pyrazole treatment led to a significant decrease in the activity of benzphetamine demethylase. 4-Iodopyrazole increased the turnover (nmol/min/nmol P-450) of EROD and PNPH by 1.5 fold each. 4-Nitropyrazole had no significant effect on any of the activities or turnover rates tested. In contrast to results with cultured chick hepatocytes, where induction was directly related to the hydrophobicity of the 4-substituent, the

---

The authors are affiliated with the Laboratory of Metabolism and Molecular Biology, Division of Intramural Clinical and Biological Research, National Institute of Alcohol Abuse and Alcoholism, 12501 Washington Avenue, Rockville, MD 20852.

Reprint requests should be sent to N. W. Cornell.

present data indicate that the process of induction *in vivo* is more complex.

INTRODUCTION

Pyrazole (Pyr) and its 4-substituted derivatives are potent inhibitors of alcohol dehydrogenase and have been proposed as agents for the treatment of alcohol toxicity.[1] However pyrazoles also alter cytochrome P-450-catalyzed drug metabolism.[2-5] For example, they induce cytochrome P-450 in cultured chick embryo hepatocytes, and tests with 8 compounds showed that induction was dependent only on the pyrazoles' hydrophobicity.[4] With rat microsomes, we observed that hydrophobicity also determined the potency of pyrazoles as ligands and inhibitors of cytochrome P-450.[6] Pyr and 4-methylpyrazole (MP) have been shown to induce the rat liver cytochrome P-450j isozyme[5] which possesses essentially all of the microsomal p-nitrophenol hydroxylase (PNPH) activity.[7] In the present study, we attempted to determine the relative effectiveness of 5 pyrazoles as inducers of rat hepatic PNPH activity *in vivo*. Since there is evidence that more than one isozyme is induced following treatment with MP,[3,5] we also measured the activities of 7-ethoxyresorufin O-deethylase (EROD) and benzphetamine N-demethylase (BPD) as indicators of cytochromes P-450$_c$ and P-450$_b$, respectively.[8] This information is important in determining potential side effects of 4-substituted pyrazoles that might be used in treatment of alcohol toxicity.

METHODS

Liver microsomes were prepared by differential centrifugation from 24-hour fasted male Wistar rats that had received 3 consecutive daily intraperitoneal injections (200 mg/kg body weight) or Pyr, MP, 4-pentylpyrazole hydrochloride (PP-HCl), all in 0.9% saline, 4-iodopyrazole (IP) in corn oil, or 4-nitropyrazole (NP) in 95% ethanol. Control rats were given comparable amounts of solvent. Microsomal protein,[9] cytochrome P-450,[10] and PNPH,[11] BPD,[12] and EROD[13] activities were measured. Data was analyzed using Student's two-sided t-test.

RESULTS AND DISCUSSION

Two of the Pyr-tested rats had stomachs bloated with undigested food, though food had been withheld for 24 hours. Because only one of the five rats treated with PP-HCl survived the treatment, no statistical significance could be placed on these measurements. Two of the four EtOH-treated and one of the NP-treated rats also died during the treatment period.

As shown in Table 1, only pyrazole caused a significant increase in liver size. This agrees with the hepatotoxic nature of this compound as described previously.[2] The content of cytochrome P-450

Table 1.
The effects of pyraxoles on rat liver weight, hepatic microsomal cytochrome P-450 content, and mixed function oxidase activities. Cytochrome P-450 content is expressed as nmol/mg of microsomal protein. Activities per mg microsomal protein (A.) and turnovers per nmol cytochrome P-450 (B.) are expressed as nmol/min for PNPH and BPD and as pmol/min for EROD. The numbers presented are the mean (and standard deviation) of determinations from n rats.

Treatment	Saline	Pyr	MP	PP-HCl	corn oil	IP	EtoH	NP
Log P		0.26	0.96	2.96		1.70		0.59
n	7	5	5	1	3	5	2	4
g liver/ 100 g b.w.	4.26 (0.34)	5.59^a (0.28)	4.65 (0.31)	4.30	4.61 (0.10)	4.61 (0.13)	4.60 (0.22)	4.94 (0.61)
cytochrome P-450	0.73 (0.17)	0.82 (0.21)	0.96 (0.22)	0.53	0.50^a (0.02)	0.50^a (0.11)	0.46^a (0.08)	0.53 (0.14)
A. Activities								
PNPH	2.09 (0.20)	4.07^a (0.82)	4.01^a (1.94)	0.48	2.44 (0.38)	3.79^a (1.61)	1.36 (0.67)	2.10 (0.56)
BPD	1.96 (0.23)	0.71^a (0.27)	2.22 (0.55)	3.50	2.32 (0.31)	1.99 (0.21)	1.85 (0.21)	2.08 (0.30)
EROD	17.8 (6.1)	19.4 (7.5)	56.7 (20.9)	134	28.2^a (0.6)	43.5^a (19.9)	47.6^a (20.7)	31.2^a (7.0)
B. Turnovers								
PNPH	3.02 (0.85)	5.23^a (1.49)	3.98 (1.29)	0.90	4.92^a (0.62)	7.45^{a,b} (1.99)	2.93 (1.46)	4.40^a (0.75)
BPD	2.87 (0.94)	0.93^a (0.44)	2.50 (1.24)	6.58	4.70^a (0.77)	4.10^a (0.72)	4.11 (0.93)	4.56 (1.59)
EROD	24.4 (5.5)	24.6 (10.7)	59.8^a (20.1)	252	57.0^a (2.0)	84.6^{a,b} (23.1)	1.05^a (48)	65.7^a (10.1)

^{a}Different from saline control at $p < 0.05$.
^{b}Different from corn oil control at $p < 0.05$.

was decreased by treatment with corn oil or EtOH, although there was no significant decrease in any of the activities measured. This suggests the deinduction of isozyme(s) other than the ones measured.

Pyr, MP, and IP significantly increased the activity of PNPH, but this induction was not correlated with the hydrophobicity of the pyrazoles as had been predicted. On the contrary, this activity was dramatically decreased by the most lipophilic compound tested, PP-HCl. Only Pyr caused a significant change in BPD, although this activity was greatly increased by PP-HCl treatment. The log of P, the octanol:water partition coefficient,[14] directly correlated with the activity ($r = 0.925$) and turnover ($r = 0.946$) of EROD in the treated groups, indicating the more lipophilic pyrazoles acted as better inducers. This is in agreement with the data of Cornell et al.[15] which showed a 48-fold induction of this activity in chick embryo hepatocytes treated with 4-hexylpyrazole.

Gross toxicity of the pyrazoles could not be correlated with any of the activities measured. Further studies are required to characterize the toxicities and to delineate the inductive responses to each pyrazole in order to identify relationships between structure and function *in vivo*.

REFERENCES

1. Blomstrand R, Ellin A, Lof A, Ostling-Wintzell H. Biological effects and metabolic interactions after chronic and acute administration of 4-methylpyrazole and ethanol to rats. Arch Biochem Biophys. 1980; 199:591-605.

2. Lieber C, Rubin E, DeCarli LM, Misra P, Gang H. Effects of pyrazoles on hepatic function. Lab Invest. 1970; 22:615-621.

3. Krikun G, Feierman DE, Cederbaum AI. Rat liver microsomal induction of the oxidation of drugs and alcohols, and sodium dodecyl sulfate-gel profiles after in vivo treatment with pyrazole or 4-methylpyrazole. J Pharm Exp Ther. 1986; 237:1012-1019.

4. Sinclair J, Cornell NW, Zaitlin L, Hansch C. Induction of cytochrome P-450 by alcohols and 4-substituted pyrazoles. Comparisons of structure-activity relationships. Biochem Pharmacol. 1986; 35:707-710.

5. Song BJ, Gelboin HV, Park SS, Yang CS, Gonzalez FJ. Complementary DNA and protein sequences of ethanol-inducible rat and human cytochrome P-450s. J Biol Chem. 1986; 261:16689-16697.

6. Marden LJ, Cornell NW, Sinclair JF, Stegeman JJ. Pyrazoles as ligands and inducers of cytochrome P-450. Fed Proc. 1987; 47:865.

7. Koop DR. Hydroxylation of p-nitrophenol by rabbit ethanol-inducible cytochrome P-450 isozyme 3a. Mol Pharmacol. 1986; 29:399-404.

8. Conney AH. Induction of microsomal cytochrome P-450. Life Sciences. 1985; 39:2493-2518.

9. Pierce Chemical Company, BCA and BCA protein Assay Reagent, Instructions 23230, 23225, 1986.

10. Omura T and Sato R. The carbon monoxide-binding pigment of liver microsomes. II. Solubilization, purification, and properties. J Biol Chem. 1964; 239:2379-2385.

11. Reinke LA and Moyer MJ. p-Nitrophenol hydroxylation: A microsomal oxidation which is highly inducible by ethanol. Drug Metab Dispos. 1985; 13:548-552.

12. Hewick D and Fouts J. Effects of storage on hepatic microsomal cytochromes and substrate-inducible difference spectra. Biochem Pharmacol. 1970; 19:457-472.

13. Prough RA, Burke MD, Mayer RT. Direct fluorometric methods for measuring mixed-function oxidase. Methods in Enzymology. 1978; 52:372-377.

14. Hansch C and Leo A. Substituents for Correlation Analysis in Chemistry and Biology. 1979; Wiley-Interscience, New York.

15. Cornell NW, Sinclair JF, Stegeman JH, Hansch C. Pyrazoles as effectors of ethanol oxidizing enzymes and inducers of cytochrome P-450. Alcohol & Alcoholism. 1987; Suppl. 1:251-255.

Structure and Regulation of the Ethanol-Inducible Cytochrome P450j

B. J. Song, PhD
R. L. Veech, MD, DPhil
S. S. Park, PhD
H. V. Gelboin, PhD
F. J. Gonzalez, PhD

SUMMARY. Specific polyclonal antisera against microsomal ethanol-inducible cytochrome P450 (P450j, P450IIE) were prepared and utilized to isolate cDNA for P450j from λgt11 cDNA libraries. The longest cDNAs encoding P450j of rat and human were completely sequenced. The rat P450j sequence was compared to those of other P450s (P450II gene family members) to determine the structural similarity. Southern-blot analysis of rat and human genomic DNAs verified that only a single gene shared extensive homology with P450j.

Cloned P450j cDNA and antibodies were used to study the expression of P450j gene during development and by various inducers as well as in pathological conditions. By combination of cDNA hybridization and immunoblot analyses, three types of P450j gene expression were observed: transcriptional activation during development; post-transcriptional activation (probably via protein stabilization) by various inducers such as pyrazole, 4-methylpyrazole, acetone, and ethanol; and mRNA stabilization in diabetic and starved animals. These three different types of P450j induction ap-

B. J. Song and R. L. Veech are affiliated with the Laboratory of Metabolism and Molecular Biology, Division of Intramural Clinical and Biological Research, National Institute on Alcohol Abuse and Alcoholism, 12501 Washington Avenue, Rockville, MD 20852. S. S. Park, H. V. Gelboin, and F. J. Gonzalez are affiliated with the Laboratory of Molecular Carcinogenesis, National Cancer Institute, National Institutes of Health, Bethesda, MD 20892.

peared to be present not only in liver but also in lung and kidney tissues.

INTRODUCTION

The cytochrome P450s, terminal components of the microsomal mixed function monooxygenase system, metabolize a variety of xenobiotics as well as endogenous substrates like steroids and prostaglandins. The multiplicity, induction and regulation of P450 genes have recently been reviewed.[1] The ethanol-inducible P450j (P450IIE1) is involved in the metabolism of nitrosamines,[2] carbon tetrachloride,[3] and certain aromatic compounds.[4] It has been shown to be induced by many structurally unrelated compounds as well as in pathophysiological conditions. In order to study the mechanism of this unique induction process and to develop specific probes in analyzing potential variations in alcohol and nitrosamine metabolism, the cDNA for P450j was isolated, characterized, and utilized.

METHODS

All the experimental methods were described in detail.[5,6,7]

RESULTS AND DISCUSSION

Specific monoclonal and polyclonal antibodies against P450j were prepared and used to isolate cDNA for P450j from λgt11 cDNA libraries. The longest cDNAs encoding P450j of both rat and human were completely sequenced and found to be related to P450s in the P450II gene family. Southern-blot analysis of rat and human genomic DNAs verified that only a single gene shared extensive homology with P450j. Cloned P450j cDNA and antibodies were used to study the regulatory mechanism of P450j expression during development and by various inducers as well as in pathological conditions. By combination of cDNA hydridization and immunoblot analyses, three types of P450j gene expression were observed: transcriptional activation during development; post-transcriptional activation (probably via protein stabilization) by various chemical inducers such as ethanol, acetone, and pyrazoles; and mRNA stabilization in diabetic and starved animals. These three different types of P450j induction appeared to be active not only in liver but also in lung and kidney tissues.

REFERENCES

1. Nebert DW, Gonzalez FJ. P450 genes; Structure, evolution, and regulation. Ann Rev Biochem. 1987; 56:945-993.

2. Yang CS, Koop DR, Wang T, Coon MJ. Immunochemical studies on the metabolism of nitrosamines by ethanol-inducible cytochrome P-450. Biochem Biophys Res Comm. 1985; 128:1007-1013.

3. English JC, Anders MW. Evidence for the metabolism of N-nitrosodimethylamine and carbon tetrachloride by a common isozyme of cytochrome P450. Drug Metab Dispos. 1985; 13:449-452.

4. Koop DR. Hydroxylation of p-nitrophenol by rabbit ethanol-inducible cytochrome P450 isozyme 3a. Mol Pharmacol. 1986; 29:399-404.

5. Song BJ, Gleboin HV, Park SS, Yang CS, Gonzalez FJ. Complementary DNA and protein sequences of ethanol-inducible rat and human P-450s: Transcriptional and post-transcriptional regulation of the rat enzyme. J Biol Chem. 1986; 261:16689-16697.

6. Song BJ, Matsunaga T, Hardwick JP, Park SS, Veech RL, Yang CS, Gelboin HV, Gonzalez FJ. Stabilization of cytochrome P450j mRNA in the diabetic rat. Mol Endocrinol. 1987; in press.

7. Ko IY, Park SS, Song BJ, Patten C, Tan Y, Hah YC, Yang CS, Gelboin HV. Monoclonal antibodies to ethanol-induced rat liver cytochrome P450 that metabolizes aniline and nitrosamines. Cancer Res. 1987; 47:3101-3109.

Epidermal Growth Factor Binding in the Presence of Ethanol

M. J. Gerhart, MS
B. Y. Reed, PhD
R. L. Veech, MD, DPhil

SUMMARY. Epidermal growth factor (EGF) is a mitogen which has been shown to stimulate maxillo-facial growth and DNA synthesis. Ethanol has been reported to inhibit cell regeneration *in vivo* and *in vitro* and to produce diminished maxillo-facial development in fetal alcohol syndrome. Recent findings from this laboratory have elucidated rapid metabolic changes in the hepatic content of some of the glycolytic intermediates resulting from injection of EGF, ethanol or EGF combined with ethanol *in vivo*. An immediate effect of EGF *in vivo* is to increase hepatic tissue content of 3-phosphoglycerate and phosphoenolpyruvate 1.2-1.3 fold when compared to saline treatment. Ethanol however causes a marked fall in the hepatic content of 3-phosphoglycerate and phosphoenolpyruvate 3.2-3.7 fold below saline treated levels. Ethanol in combination with EGF decreases hepatic values for 3-phosphoglycerate and phosphoenolpyruvate 2.0-2.3 fold from saline treated, but elevates the content of phosphoenolpyruvate 1.6 fold over ethanol treatment alone. Such metabolite changes occurring with ethanol treatment have been attributed alternately to redox shifts or to membrane perturbations. We wished to determine whether dimunition of 3-phosphoglycerate and or phosphoenolpyruvate below certain levels perhaps critically necessary for normal mitogenic action of EGF was due in this case to ethanol effects of binding of EGF to the cell membrane.

The authors are affiliated with the Laboratory of Metabolism and Molecular Biology, Division of Intramural Clinical and Biological Research, National Institute on Alcohol Abuse and Alcoholism, 12501 Washington Avenue, Rockville, MD 20852.

Reprint requests should be sent to M. J. Gerhart.

INTRODUCTION

Epidermal growth factor (EGF) is a mitogen which has been shown to stimulate maxillo-facial growth and DNA synthesis.[1,2] Ethanol has been reported to inhibit cell regeneration *in vivo* and *in vitro*[3,4] and to produce diminished maxillo-facial development in fetal alcohol syndrome.[5] Recent findings from this laboratory have shown rapid metabolic changes in the hepatic content of some of the glycolytic intermediates resulting from injection of EGF, ethanol or EGF combined with ethanol *in vivo*.[6] Specifically, an immediate effect of EGF *in vivo* is to increase hepatic tissue content of 3-phosphoglycerate and phosphoenolpyruvate 1.3 fold when compared to saline treatment. Ethanol in combination with EGF decreases hepatic values for 3-phosphoglycerate and phosphoenolpyruvate 2.0-2.3 fold from saline treated, but elevates the content of phosphoenolpyruvate 1.6 fold over ethanol treatment alone. Such metabolite changes occurring with ethanol treatment have been attributed to redox shifts.[7] Alternately dimunition of EGF induced metabolite changes seen with ethanol treatment could also be a secondary result of decreased EGF binding.[8] We wished to determine whether ethanol effects the binding of EGF to the cell membrane.

METHODS AND MATERIALS

A431 cells (ATTC), derived from human epidermoid carcinoma of the vulva, were grown to 80% confluence in 60mm Falcon plastic dishes using 4 ml of Dulbecco's MEM supplemented with 1000 U/ml penicillin, 100 ug/ml streptomycin and 10% fetal calf serum (DMEM complete). Assay procedures were as described elsewhere[9] with the following modifications. Binding media containing no ethanol, 25mM ethanol or 100mM ethanol was added to the appropriate dish and each dish was incubated 20 minutes at 37°C. Ethanol concentrations were those used in the previous study[6] or those found to be maximally inhibitory of EGF action.[4] Each dish was then brought to 1.6 nmolar EGF[I125] (GIBCO,BTI) and allowed to incubate at 37°C for 5 minutes. Three washes with ice cold Hank's plus .1% BSA was followed by an additional 3 washes with Hank's minus BSA to remove any remaining calf serum. After solubilization the 1 N NaOH solution was pipetted into a tube with 2 additional washes of 1 ml each of Hank's and counted in a gamma counter. Lowry protein determinations were done and statistics were calculated using the student's t-test.

RESULTS AND CONCLUSIONS

For each concentration of ethanol tested the rate of binding was 13ng of EGF per milligram of protein. We conclude that treatment of A431 cells with ethanol did not alter the ability of these cells to bind EGF to its membrane receptor.

REFERENCES

1. Cohen S. Isolation of a mouse submaxillary gland protein accelerating incisor eruption and eyelid opening in the newborn animal. J Biol Chem. 1962; 237:1555-1562.

2. Carpenter G, Cohen S. Human epidermal growth factor and the proliferation of human fibroblasts. J Cell Physiol. 1976a; 88:227.

3. Poso R, Poso H, Vaananen H, Salaspuro M. Inhibition of macromolecules by ethanol in regenerating rat liver. Adv Exptl Biol Med. 1980; 132:551-560.

4. Carter EA, Wands JR. Ethanol inhibits hormone stimulated hepatocyte DNA synthesis. BBRC 1985; 128(2):767-774.

5. Ouellette EM, Rosett HL, Rosman NP, Weiner L. Adverse effects on offspring of maternal alcohol abuse during pregnancy. N Engl J Med. 1977; 297:528-530.

6. Gerhart MJ, Reed BY, Veech RL. Ethanol Inhibits Some of the Early Effects of Epidermal Growth Factor *in vivo*. Alcohol: Clin Exper Res. 1988; 12(1):116-118.

7. Veech RL, Guynn R, Veloso D. The time-course of the effects of ethanol on the redox and phosphorylation states of rat liver. Biochem J. 1972; 127:387-397.

8. Bannister MB, Losowsky MS. Cell Receptors and Ethanol. Alcohol: Clin Exper Res. 1986; 10(6):50S-54S.

9. Carpenter G. Binding Assays for Epidermal Growth Factor. J. Cell Biol. 1976; 71:159.

Phosphorus-31 Nuclear Magnetic Resonance Spectroscopic Study of the Canine Pancreas: Applications to Acute Alcoholic Pancreatitis

Nathan Janes, PhD
Jeffrey A. Clemens, MD
Jerry D. Glickson, PhD
John L. Cameron, MD

SUMMARY. The first nuclear magnetic resonance spectroscopic study of the canine pancreas is described. Both in-vivo, ex-vivo protocols and nmr observables are discussed. The stability of the ex-vivo preparation based on the nmr observables is established for at least four hours. The spectra obtained from the in-vivo and ex-vivo preparations exhibited similar metabolite ratios, further validating the model. Metabolite levels were unchanged by a 50% increase in perfusion rate. Only trace amounts of phosphocreatine were observed either in the intact gland or in extracts. Acute alcoholic pancreatitis was mimicked by free fatty acid infusion. Injury resulted in

Jeffrey A. Clemens and John L. Cameron are affiliated with the Department of Surgery and Nathan Janes and Jerry D. Glickson are affiliated with the Department of Radiology, Johns Hopkins University, School of Medicine, Baltimore, MD 21205. In addition, Nathan Janes is affiliated with the National Institute on Alcohol Abuse and Alcoholism, 12501 Washington Avenue, Rockville, MD 20852. Reprint requests should be addressed to him.

This research was supported in part by NIH 5R01 AM 32435-02 (JAC, JLC) and NRSA 1F32 AA05247 (NJ).

The authors would like to thank VP Chacko for many helpful discussions and Fred Gilliam for expert technical assistance. They would also like to thank Dr. JD Glickson, the JHMI NMR Center, and Varian Instruments for support.

hyperamylasemia, edema (weight gain), increased hematocrit and perfusion pressure, and depressed levels of high energy phosphates.

Clinical pancreatitis is diagnosed in 0.9 to 9.5% of alcoholic patients, while pathological evidence of pancreatitis is observed in 17 to 45% of alcoholics.[1] A review of over 5000 cases of acute pancreatitis attributed 55% to alcohol use.[1] The pathogenesis of the disease is yet poorly understood and treatment, therefore, is primarily symptomatic and supportive, lacking a proven therapeutic regimen.[1]

In order to better understand the cellular events leading to injury, we have developed a protocol for the first phosphorus-31 nuclear magnetic resonance (nmr) spectroscopic investigation of the in-vivo and ex-vivo canine pancreas in order to characterize the energetic status of the gland. As approximately 95-98% of the gland mass is devoted to exocrine function, of which 90% consists of acinar cells,[2] this investigation is predominantly reflective of the properties of intact, functional acinar cells. Protein synthesis, transport, secretion, and retention are energy dependent processes.[3,4] The turnover rate of the high energy phosphate pool is 23 seconds.[3] To our knowledge, there have been two brief reports of P-31 nmr spectra of the perfused rat pancreas,[5,6] none of the in-vivo system.

METHODS

The blood-perfused canine pancreas preparation is diagrammed in Figure 1A, and described in detail elsewhere.[7] Blood gases, serum amylase, hematocrit, and glucose were recorded hourly, and the gland was weighed before and after the protocol. The in-vivo measurements were performed on an anesthetized dog (nembutal 30mg/kg). A solenoidal nmr coil was positioned around the tail of the pancreas following splenectomy, and the abdomen closed. Cardiac sufficiency was monitored via cannulation of the femoral artery.

NMR spectra were obtained on a Varian VXR console and Oxford Instrument 4.7T horizontal 33cm bore magnet, operating at 80.9 MHz for phosphorus. Spectra were obtained using a homemade 3 cm surface coil on the uncinate process, or a solenoidal coil

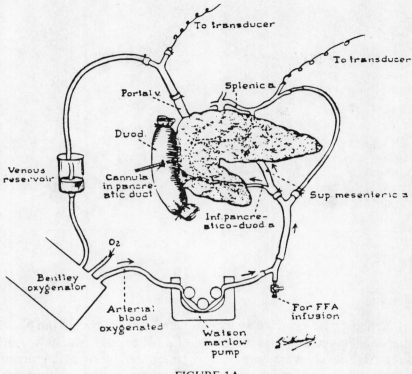

FIGURE 1A

around the tail. A capillary of methylene diphosphonate served as reference. Spectra were obtained using a one pulse sequence, without proton decoupling, at intervals of 1 second or 20 seconds.

RESULTS

A typical spectrum of the normoxic canine pancreas is shown in Figure 1B. Under partially saturating conditions, very good signal to noise could be obtained in less than ten minutes. The nucleoside triphosphates (presumably ATP) are predominantly complexed to magnesium, based on the chemical shift difference between the α and β resonances (8.7 ppm).[8] The resonance position of the inor-

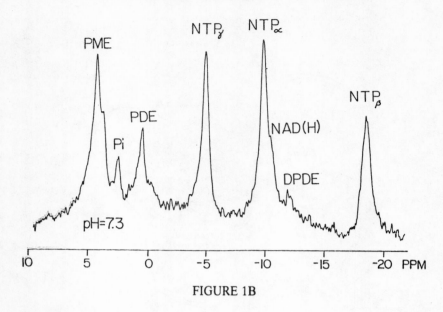

FIGURE 1B

ganic phosphate (which may include small contributions from blood diphosphoglycerate) was indicative of a pH of approximately 7.3.[8] Free ADP levels were undetectably small. Perchloric acid extracts were used to confirm the presence of glycerophosphocholine and glycerophosphoethanolamine in the phosphodiester region, based on titration of extracts as observed by nmr.[8] The energetic stability of the normoxid gland was established for four hours.

It has recently been reported[5] that the isolated rat pancreas preparation is partially ischemic. Increases in the flow rate by 50% in this preparation caused no detectable spectral perturbations. A comparison of the fully relaxed spectra from the in-vivo and ex-vivo pancreas are shown in Figure 2A and show no evidence of inadequate perfusion in the ex-vivo preparation, and the close similarity between the two reinforce the suitability of the ex-vivo model. Furthermore, the NTP/Pi ratios compare very favorably with those reported for the perfused rat pancreas (even at high flow rates). Only trace levels of phosphocreatine were observed when duodenal contamination was avoided, in the ex-vivo, in-vivo, and biopsy extract

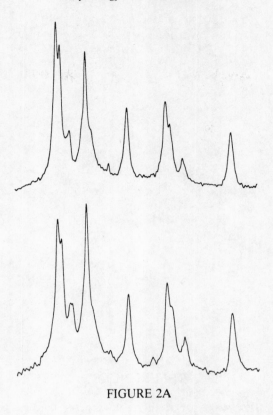

FIGURE 2A

spectra. This is consistent with earlier results,[3,6,9] although there are some exceptions.[5,10]

Shown in Figure 2B are spectra recorded after infusion of 0.3 ml oleic acid, a model for acute alcoholic pancreatitis based on the associated hyperlipidemia.[7] The model produces edematous pancreatitis resulting in weight gain, hyperamylasemia, increased perfusion pressure, increased hematocrit and hemoglobin serum levels, in conjunction with declines in the NTP levels as shown.

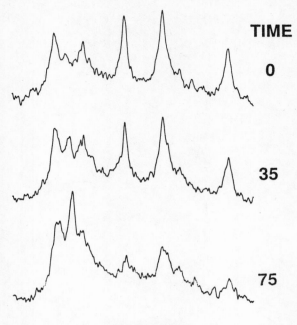

FIGURE 2B

REFERENCES

1. Ranson JHC. Acute pancreatitis: pathogenesis, outcome and treatment. Clin Gastroent. 1984; 13:843-863; and references therein.

2. Tompkins RK, Traverso LW. The exocrine cells. In: Keynes WM, Keith RG, eds. The pancreas. New York: Appleton-Century-Crofts, 1981.

3. Bauduin H, Colin M, Dumont JE. Energy sources for protein synthesis and enzymatic secretion in rat pancreas in vitro. Biochim Biophys Acta. 1969; 174:722-733.

4. Case RM. Synthesis, intracellular transport and discharge of exportable proteins in the pancreatic acinar cell and other cells. Biol Rev. 1978; 53:211-354; and references therein.

5. Kaplan O, Kushnir T, Navon G. P-31 nmr study of perfused rat pancreas and experimental pancreatitis. Soc Magn Reson Med, Book of abstracts, Fifth Meeting. 1986; 3:906-907.

6. Komabayashi T, Watanabe K, Izawa T, Tsuboi M. ^{31}P-nmr studies of energy metabolites in rat pancreas treated with trypsin inhibitor. Res Comm Chem Path Pharm. 1986; 53:249-252.

7. Sanfey H. Bulkley GB, Cameron JL. The pathogenesis of acute pancreati-

tis: The source and role of oxygen-derived free radicals in three different experimental models. Ann Surg. 1985; 201:633-639.

8. Gadian DG. Nuclear Magnetic Resonance and its applications to living systems. New York: Oxford University Press, 1982; and references therein.

9. Thorn VW, Liemann F, Hirsch R, Straub K. Metabolitstatus, RNS-gehalt und ausscheidungsfunktion des katzenpancreas unter infusion von gewebshormonen und ischamischer belastung. Arzneimittel-Forsch, 1967; 12:1469-1472.

10. Becker H, Vinten-Johansen J, Buckberg GD, Bugyi HI. Correlation of pancreatic blood flow and high-energy phosphates during experimental pancreatitis. Eur Surg Res. 1982; 14:203-210.

The Effect of Alcohol Inhalation on the Cardiovascular State of the Rat

John W. Karanian, PhD
Norman Salem, Jr., PhD

SUMMARY. Rats were exposed to alcohol vapors by an inhalation technique and blood pressure and its reactivity and platelet aggregation were measured. *Acute* exposure to alcohol levels which produced moderate blood alcohol concentration (BAC) was associated with increased vascular production of prostacyclin (PGI_2) and plasma catecholamines, whereas platelet production of thromboxane (TXA_2) decreased. Blood pressure is elevated in these animals, however, the platelet aggregating and pressor effects of noradrenaline (NE) were decreased. *Chronic* exposure to high BAC is associated with a dramatic reduction in vascular and platelet prostaglandin (PG) production and a marked increase in plasma catecholamine levels. Platelet aggregation decreased in these animals, however, the pressor effect of TXA_2 and NE was significantly increased. The fatty acid precursors to PG were reduced by 50% in the lipid extracts of these preparations. These findings suggest that alterations in fatty acid metabolism may lead to a functional deficiency in PG production from dependent rats. Qualitative differences may exist between acute and chronic exposure with respect to the cardiovascular state. Locally produced PG and circulating catecholamines may mediate alcohol-induced alterations in vascular smooth muscle tone and platelet aggregation.

INTRODUCTION

Epidemiologic studies on alcoholics and the general population indicate a strong relationship between the level of ethanol consump-

The authors are affiliated with the Section of Analytical Chemistry, Laboratory of Clinical Studies, Division of Intramural Clinical and Biological Research, National Institute on Alcohol Abuse and Alcoholism, NIH Clinical Center, Bldg. 10, Rm. 3C212, Bethesda, MD 20892.

Reprint requests should be sent to John W. Karanian.

tion and blood pressure elevation, myocardial, and cerebral infarct and vasospasm.[1] Ethanol-induced changes in blood pressure, vasoreactivity and platelet aggregation may have common etiologies which include the disruption of prostaglandin metabolism and catecholamine secretion. Alcohol has been shown to markedly alter w-6 fatty acid levels, prostaglandin (PG) metabolism, and catecholamine levels in the cardiovascular system.[2] Prostaglandins such as prostacyclin (PGI_2) and thromboxane (TXA_2), and catecholamines such as epinephrine (E) and norepinephrine (NE) are active in the cardiovascular system and may play a role in the pathophysiology associated with ethanol consumption. Using our automated apparatus for precise control of inhalation chamber alcohol vapor and blood alcohol concentrations, the effects of a range of alcohol doses on vascular tone and reactivity, platelet aggregation, fatty acid content, prostaglandin production and plasma catecholamine levels were determined in the rat.[3]

METHODS

Male rats (300-350g) were exposed to alcohol vapors for an acute (1-day) or chronic period (7-day or 14-day) before *in vitro* measurement of fatty acid levels, prostaglandin production and platelet aggregation, and measurement of plasma catecholamine levels and vasoreactivity *in vivo*. Blood alcohol levels (BAL) were maintained at $> 120mg\%$ and monitored throughout the exposure period via an enzyme assay. Subjects were removed from inhalation chambers following the vapor exposure period, and a Bligh-Dyer lipid extraction was performed on various tissues for determination of fatty acid content.[4] PG levels were determined by RIA in similarly treated animals.[5] In addition, the ventral tail artery was cannulated and rats were harnessed and tethered to a swivel to which the cannula was connected. The intraarterial line was routed through ports to pressure transducers on the outside of the chamber. The pressure transducers were connected to an eight-channel pen recorder via universal amplifiers. Graded pressor-response curves for both NE and a TXA_2-agonist (U46619) were generated.[6] Blood samples for plasma catecholamine determination were obtained from the cannula on the outside of the inhalation chamber.

RESULTS

Effect of alcohol exposure on blood pressure, plasma norepinephrine (NE) levels and its pressor response: Mean arterial blood pressure was elevated 15% in alcohol exposed (1-day) as compared to alcohol naive rats. Plasma NE levels were elevated in the same population of rats by 291% (a comparable increase in plasma E was observed). The pressor response to exogenously administered NE (400ng) was 15% lower in the alcohol exposed rat. In comparison, after a 7-day exposure to alcohol (mean BAL < 170mg%), mean arterial blood pressure was not significantly elevated although plasma NE levels were mildly elevated (51%)(increases in plasma E levels were comparable). A hyperreactivity to exogenously administered NE was observed in these animals; 22% and 25% increases were observed after a 7- and 14-day exposure to alcohol, respectively.

Effect of alcohol exposure on platelet aggregation: Platelets obtained from alcohol exposed rats were less aggregable to ADP (3uM, 16%) and arachidonic acid (40uM, 37%) after as little as a 1-day exposure to alcohol. After a longer term exposure to alcohol (7-day). ADP and arachidonate-induced aggregation decreased by 38% and 77%, respectively.

Effect of alcohol exposure on platelet TXA$_2$ production: A 1-day exposure to alcohol decreased the capacity of platelets to produce TXB$_2$ by 44% as measured by radioimmunoassay. After a 7-day exposure to alcohol vapors, a 78% decrease was observed in thromboxane levels.

Effect of alcohol exposure on the pressor response to a TXA$_2$-agonist: The pressor response to an exogenously administered TXA$_2$-mimic (U46619) (1600ng) was not significantly altered after a 1-day alcohol exposure period. However, longer alcohol exposure (7- or 14-day) was associated with a marked hyperreactivity to the pressor effects of thromboxane.

Effect of alcohol exposure on vascular PGI$_2$ production: Vascular production of PGI$_2$ (the stable non-enzymatic breakdown product 6-keto-PGF$_{1a}$ measured by radioimmunoassay)increased by more than 100% in both the rat aorta and a cerebral microvascular preparation after a 1-day exposure to alcohol. Following a longer exposure period (7- or 14-days) aortic PGI$_2$ production decreased by 48%

whereas PGI_2 levels in the cerebral microvasculature preparation were unchanged.

Effect of alcohol exposure on w-6 fatty acid content in cardiovascular and other tissues: The proportion of w-6 fatty acids in the total lipid extract of aorta did not change following a 1-day exposure to alcohol, however, after a 7- or 14-day exposure, arachidonic acid (20:4) levels decreased markedly (50%). A similar decrease was observed for dihomogammalinolenic acid (20:3), the arachidonate precursor. In addition, 20:4 content in both the platelet and liver decreased after a 7-day alcohol exposure period. The content of 20:4 in the total lipid extracts of brain and heart was not significantly changed following the longer exposure to alcohol.

SUMMARY AND CONCLUSION

Acute exposure to alcohol was associated with elevated blood pressure. The elevation in blood pressure correlated strongly with a marked increase in plasma catecholamine levels. However, vascular reactivity to NE and platelet aggregation decreased in acutely exposed rats. An associated increase in the vasodilator/platelet anti-aggregator, PGI_2 and decrease in the vasoconstrictor/platelet aggregator, TXA_2 may partially explain decreased vasoreactivity and platelet aggregation. The result of an increased PGI_2/TXA_2 ratio may be a shift towards a vasodilatory/platelet anti-aggregatory state and could in part explain epidemiological evidence that moderate ethanol consumption is associated with a low incidence of atherosclerotic disease.[7]

Chronic alcohol exposure did not significantly alter blood pressure although plasma catecholamine levels were mildly elevated. A marked vascular hyperreactivity to both NE and the TXA_2-agonist was observed in alcohol-dependent rats. These findings may have clinical implications for human alcoholics and in the analyses of cardiovascular risk factors in patients with hypertensive and vasospastic disorders.

The decrease in platelet aggregation correlated strongly with decreased TXB_2 production. The capacity to produce prostaglandins generally decreased with longterm alcohol exposure and was associated with as much as a 50% decrease in the proportion of their fatty acid precursor, arachidonic acid. Alcohol-induced changes in fatty acid and prostaglandin levels were first observed in the platelet (1-day) and then the vasculature (7-day). The heart and brain were more resistant to alcohol-induced depletion of fatty acids and the capacity to produce prostaglandins.

Our findings are consistent with the hypotheses that increased mobilization of arachidonic acid together with inhibition of its biosynthesis[8] may ultimately lead to a decrease in the capacity to produce prostaglandins in the vasculature and platelets of alcohol-dependent rats. Although chronic alcohol exposure is associated with decreased prostaglandin production, their basal levels in the cardiovascular system may not be of physiological significance. Acute alcohol exposure produces qualitatively different prostaglandin/catecholamine profiles compared to chronic exposure and may therefore produce qualitatively different effects on the cardiovascular state.

REFERENCES

1. Taylor JR. Alcohol and strokes. New Engl J Med 1982; 306:1111.

2. Karanian JW, Salem N Jr. Interactions of alcohol and prostanoids in the vascular system: Implications for cardiovascular disease. In: Gallo L, ed. Cardiovascular Disease. Plenum Press, 1987; 35:299-321.

3. Karanian JW, Yergey JL, Lister RL, Linnoila M, Salem N Jr. Characterization of an automated apparatus for precise control of inhalation chamber ethanol vapor and blood ethanol concentration. Alcoholism Clin Exp Res 1986; 10:16-22.

4. Bligh EG, Dyer WJ. A rapid method of total lipid extraction and purification. Can J Biochem Physiol 1959; 37:911-7.

5. Karanian JW, D'Souza NB, Salem N Jr. The effect of ethanol on prostacyclin and thromboxane A_2 synthesis in rat aortic rings in vitro. Prostaglandins Leukotrienes Med 1985; 20:175-86.

6. Karanian JW, D'Souza NB, Salem N Jr. The effect of chronic ethanol inhalation on blood pressure and the pressor response to noradrenaline and the thromboxane-mimic U46619. Life Sci 1986; 39:1245-55.

7. Doll R. Prospects for prevention. Br J Med 1983; 286:445-53.

8. Nervi AM, Peluffo RO, Brenner RR, Leiken AI. Effect of ethanol administration on fatty acid desaturation. Lipids 1980; 15:263-8.

Acute Effect of Intragastric Ethanol Administration on Plasma Levels of Stress Hormones

A. B. Thiagarajan, MD
I. N. Mefford, PhD
R. L. Eskay, PhD

SUMMARY. We have previously demonstrated that single-dose ethanol administration enhanced plasma levels of ACTH, β-endorphin, corticosterone (CS) and catecholamines. Since the secretion of proopiomelanocortin-derived peptides (e.g., ACTH, β-endorphin) can be influenced by catecholamines and vasopressin in addition to the primary physiological regulator, corticotrophin-releasing hormone, we have attempted to determine whether or not the ethanol-induced activation of the hypothalamic-pituitary-adrenal axis (HPAA) could in part be mediated via either epinephrine or vasopressin (AVP) secretion. The selective neutralization of AVP through the administration of AVP antiserum failed to block the ethanol-induced secretion of either ACTH or CS. In addition, adrenal demedullation did not significantly attenuate the ethanol-induced increase of ACTH and CS. It would appear that neither adrenal medulla-derived epinephrine nor median eminence-derived AVP mediates ethanol's activation of the HPAA.

INTRODUCTION

Numerous reports indicate that ethanol activates the hypothalamic-pituitary-adrenal (HPA) or stress axis.[1,2] Single-dose ethanol

A. B. Thiagarajan and R. L. Eskay are affiliated with the Laboratory of Clinical Studies, Division of Intramural Clinical and Biological Research, National Institute on Alcohol Abuse and Alcoholism, NIH Clinical Center, Bldg. 10, Rm. 3C218, Bethesda, MD 20892. I. N. Mefford is affiliated with the Section of Clinical Pharmacology, Laboratory of Clinical Studies, National Institute of Mental Health, Bethesda, MD 20892.
Reprint requests should be sent to R. L. Eskay.

administration results in increased secretion of adrenocorticotropin (ACTH) and glucocorticoids in both humans and animals. There is also considerable evidence that chronic alcohol consumption disrupts the HPA axis, which is typified by elevated glucocorticoids.[3,4] A complete understanding of the mechanism of ethanol's action on the HPA axis is currently lacking, although a recent report demonstrates that the primary physiological regulator of ACTH secretion, namely corticotropin releasing hormone (CRH), is an essential mediator of ethanol-induced ACTH release *in vivo*.[5] Since the regulation of ACTH release *in vivo* and *in vitro* is modulated by multiple endogenous factors (e.g., vasopressin, angiotensin II, catecholamines) in addition to CRH, the present study was undertaken to determine the possible role of median-eminence vasopressin and adrenomedullary catecholamines in mediating the enhanced secretion of proopiomelanocortin-derived peptides (e.g., ACTH, beta-endorphin, alpha-MSH) following acute ethanol administration.

METHODS

Adult male Sprague-Dawley rats (275-300 gm) were used in all studies. Animals were housed in individual cages and maintained on a 12 hr light/dark cycle (lights on 0600; lights off 1800) and permitted free access to food and water. Both experimental and control groups were implanted with indwelling gastric cannula one week prior to experiments. Following cannulation, animals were handled at least once a day for 4-7 days before each experiment. Blood was obtained by decapitation for plasma peptides (ACTH, alpha-MSH and beta-endorphin) and corticosterone determinations. Plasma catecholamines were determined in blood samples obtained via an indwelling jugular cannula, which was implanted 24 hrs prior to each experiment. Twelve percent ethanol in 0.9% NaCl was administered through the gastric cannula at a dose of 4 gm/kg body weight to the experimental groups, whereas, control groups received an equal volume of 0.9% NaCl. Plasma peptide and corticosterone levels were obtained by routine radioimmunoassay[6] and plasma catecholamines were determined by high performance liquid chromatography.[7] Blood ethanol levels ranged from 240-280 mg/100 ml throughout the 7.5 to 60 min post-ethanol intubation period. All experimental results are expressed as Mean ± S.E.M., unless otherwise indicated.

RESULTS AND DISCUSSION

The intragastric infusion of a moderately high dose of ethanol into naive rats resulted in a rapid and substantial increase in the release of stress hormones, as summarized in Table 1. ACTH and corticosterone were significantly elevated over basal at 7.5 min and remained elevated even after 60 min. Although not shown, immunoreactive β-endorphin/β-lipotopin, which is derived from both the anterior and intermediate lobes of the pituitary gland, as well as alpha-MSH which is of only intermediate lobe origin, were also elevated. In parallel with the observed ACTH and corticosterone

Table 1. Acute Effects Of Intragastric Ethanol Administration On The Release
Of Stress Hormones In The Rat

Time*	ACTH	Cs	Time*	Epi	Norepi
7.5	572** ± 114	229 ± 16	15	550 ± 71	229 ± 44
15	329 ± 66	202 ± 15	30	773 ± 223	212 ± 31
60	391 ± 47	368 ± 19	60	105 ± 13	179 ± 42

*-Represents time in minutes after ethanol(4 gm/kg body wt) administration. Blood ethanol levels ranged from 240-280 mg/100 ml throughout the sampling time.

**-Values represent the Mean±S.E.M of the percent increase over basal(100%); 10-15 animals were used for each treatment group.

Abbreviations: Adrenocorticotropic hormone(ACTH); Corticosterone(Cs); Epinephrine(Epi); Norepinephrine(Norepi).

changes, ethanol treatment enhanced plasma catecholamine levels 2 to 7 fold (Table 1). Epinephrine levels were augmented 5-7 fold within 15 min and returned to basal by 60 min, whereas, norepinephrine levels increased only 2 fold and remained elevated for the duration of the experiment. In an attempt to better understand the mechanism of action of ethanol's activation of the HPA axis, rats were pretreated with either a ganglion blocker (pentolinium, 5 mg/kg body wt) 5 min before ethanol administration or were bilaterally adrenodemedullectomized two weeks prior to the ethanol infusion. Neither procedure, which effectively eliminated the ethanol-induced surge of catecholamines, resulted in a significant attenuation of the ethanol induced secretion of ACTH or corticosterone. Furthermore, the infusion of 250 microliters of a high-titer vasopressin antiserum,[6] which effectively removed circulating systemic vasopressin and should have captured any ethanol-induced, median-eminence-derived release of vasopressin into the hypophysial portal blood, failed to block activation of the HPA axis. In summary, neither plasma catecholamines nor the possible enhanced secretion of vasopressin appear to play a significant role in mediating ethanol's activation of the HPA axis.

REFERENCES

1. Ellis FW. Effect of ethanol on plasma corticosterone levels. J Pharm Exp Ther 1966; 153:121-7.

2. Redei E, Branch BJ, Taylor AN. Direct effect of ethanol on ACTH release *in vitro*. J. Pharm Exp Ther 1986; Vol 273(1):59-64.

3. Smals AG, Kloppenberg PW, Njo KT et al. Alcohol induced Cushings Syndrome. Br Med J 1976; 1297.

4. Paton A. Alcohol induced pseudo-Cushingoid Syndrome. Br Med J 1976; 1298.

5. Rivier C, Bruhn T, Vale W. Effect of ethanol on the hypothalamic-pituitary-adrenal axis in the rat: Role of corticotropin-releasing-factor. J Pharm Exp Ther 1984; Vol 229 (1):127-31.

6. Dave JR, Rubinstein N, Eskay RL. Evidence that beta-endorphin binds to specific receptors to in rat peripheral tissues and stimulates the adenylate-cyclase-adenosine 3'5'-monophosphate system. Endocrinology 1985; 117:1389-96.

7. Mefford IN, Ota M, Stipetic M, Singleton W. Application of a novel cation exchange reagent, Igepon T-77(N-methyl Oleoyl Taurate), to microbore separation of alumina extracts of catecholamines from cerebrospinal fluid, plasma, urine, and brain tissue with amperometric detection. J Chromatogr Biomed Applic, 1987; 420:241-251.

Regulation of Vasopressin and Oxytocin Synthesis in Anterior Pituitary and Peripheral Tissues

J. R. Dave, PhD
S. G. Culp, BS
L. Liu, MS
B. Tabakoff, PhD
P. L. Hoffman, PhD

SUMMARY. Recent studies have demonstrated the presence of immunoreactive oxytocin (OT) and vasopressin (VP), OT and VP receptors and physiological functions for these two hormones in a variety of peripheral tissues, including anterior pituitary gland. The objectives of this study were to determine if (i) OT and VP genes are expressed in rat testis and anterior pituitary gland and (ii) if osmotic stimulation known to modify the regulation of OT and VP genes in hypothalamus, would modify the expression of these genes in rat testis and anterior pituitary gland. Using oligonucleotide probes (courtesy of Drs. M. Brownstein and W. Scott Young, NIMH) corresponding to the VP gene or OT gene and specific fractions of human OT and VP genes (courtesy of Dr. J. Battey, NCI) subcloned in the pGEM-3 riboprobe system, and Northern blot and slot blot techniques, OT and VP mRNAs were found in rat testis and anterior pituitary gland. When adult male rats (SD) were either deprived of drinking water or offered 2% salt solution as a sole source of drinking fluid for 72 hrs, both OT and VP mRNA levels were increased in hypothalamus, anterior pituitary gland and testis. Our data suggest that testis and anterior pituitary gland could also be sites of synthesis

The authors are affiliated with the Division of Intramural Clinical and Biological Research, National Institute on Alcohol Abuse and Alcoholism, 12501 Washington Avenue, Rockville, MD 20852.

Reprint requests should be sent to J. R. Dave.

of OT and VP and that the same stimulus may regulate these genes in various tissues.

Recent studies have demonstrated the presence of immunoreactive oxytocin (OT) and vasopressin (VP), OT and VP receptors and physiological functions for these two hormones in a variety of peripheral tissues, including anterior pituitary gland and male reproductive tract of several species. The demonstration of very high (approximately 100-fold higher than circulating levels) concentrations of OT and VP in the testis, and release of high concentrations of VP in the media of cultured anterior pituitary cells have suggested that these tissues may represent a possible peripheral source of these hormones. The objectives of this study were to determine if (i) OT and VP genes are expressed in rat testis and anterior pituitary gland and (ii) if osmotic stimulation, known to modify the regulation of OT and VP genes in hypothalamus, would modify the expression of these genes in rat testis and anterior pituitary gland.

Adult male rats (SD) were either deprived of drinking water or offered 2% salt solutions as a sole source of drinking fluid for 72 hrs, sacrificed by decapitation and various tissues and trunk blood were collected. The hypothalamus, anterior pituitary gland and testes were used for total nucleic acid isolation by the SET-PK method[1] and plasma, hypothalamus, anterior and neurointermediate lobes of the pituitary gland and testis were processed for quantitation of peptides by specific radioimmunoassays.

Using oligonucleotide probes corresponding to the VP gene or OT gene,[2] specific fractions of human OT and VP genes[3] subcloned in the pGEM-3 riboprobe system, and Northern blot and slot blot techniques, OT and VP mRNAs were detected in rat hypothalamus, testis and anterior pituitary gland. The osmotic manipulations produced an increase in circulating levels of OT and VP and a decrease in stored contents of these peptides in the neurointermediate lobe of the pituitary gland, consistent with many other reports. No significant change in the hypothalamic content of the hormones was noted in treated animals. As presented in Figure 1, the treatments increased both OT and VP mRNA levels in hypothalamus, anterior pituitary gland and testis.

While the observations in hypothalamus are consistent with find-

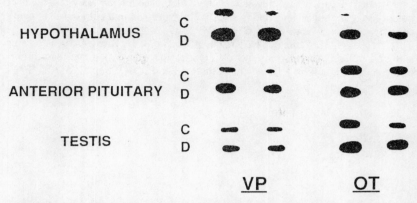

HYPOTHALAMUS C D

ANTERIOR PITUITARY C D

TESTIS C D

VP **OT**

FIGURE 1. Demonstration that water deprivation of adult male rats for 72 hrs increased oxytocin (OT) and vasopressin (VP) mRNA levels in the hypothalamus, anterior pituitary gland and testis. The slot blots were hybridized with ^{32}P-labeled oligonucleotide probes, as described in an earlier study.[1] The amount of total RNA applied is approximately the same in control (C) or water-deprived (D) groups. The size of OT or VP mRNAs, as judged by the Northern blots (data not shown), were slightly different in various tissues.

ings reported by others, this study reports, for the first time, the presence of OT and VP mRNA in rat anterior pituitary gland. Our data extend a previous report of VP and OT mRNA in the testis of the Brattleboro rat,[4] and support the hypothesis that testis and anterior pituitary gland could be sites of synthesis of OT and VP. Furthermore, our data suggest that the same stimuli may regulate these genes in various tissues, although measurement of peptide levels is also necessary.

REFERENCES

1. Dave, J.R., L.E. Eiden, J.W. Karanian & R.L. Eskay. 1986. Ethanol exposure decreases pituitary CRF binding, adenylate cyclase activity, pro-opiomelanocortin biosynthesis, and plasma β-endorphin levels in rats. Endocrinology. 118:280-286.
2. Young, W.S., E. Mezey & R.E. Siegel. 1986. Vasopressin and oxytocin mRNAs in adrenalectomized and Brattleboro rats: analysis by quantitative *in situ* hybridization histochemistry. Mol. Brain Res. 1:231-241.

3. Sausville, E., D. Carney & J. Battey. 1986. The human vasopressin gene is linked to the oxytocin gene and is selectively expressed in a cultured lung cancer cell line. J. Biol. Chem. 260:10236-10241.

4. Ivell, R., H. Schmale, B. Krisch, P. Nahke & D. Richter. 1986. Expression of a mutant vasopressin gene: differential polyadenylation and read-through of the mRNA 3′ end in a frame-shift mutant. The EMBO Journal. 5:971-977.

Discovery of Novel Brain Lipoxygenase Products Formed from Docosahexaenoic Acid (22:6w3)

T. Shingu, MD, PhD
J. W. Karanian, PhD
H. Y. Kim, PhD
J. A. Yergey, PhD
N. Salem, Jr., PhD

SUMMARY. It is known that alcohol exposure leads to a decline in brain docosahexaenoate (22:6w3). We hypothesized that alcohol could stimulate the metabolism of this polyunsaturated fatty acid to bioactive products. Several oxidized products of 22:6w3 were indeed observed when rat brain homogenate was incubated with ^{14}C22:6w3 *in vitro*. A similar group of metabolites was formed *in vivo* from ^{14}C-22:6w3 injected into the lateral ventricle. These metabolites were characterized by thermospray- and GC/MS as well as by the synthesis of standards using purified enzymes. Platelet lipoxygenase also proved useful in identifying one of the brain metabolites and served as a source of enzyme for preparative studies. Their physiological effects on smooth muscle tone and platelet aggregation will be presented.

INTRODUCTION

It is known that alcohol exposure leads to a decline in central nervous system brain docosahexaenoate (22:6w3)[1] which is the ma-

---

The authors are affiliated with the Section on Analytical Chemistry, Laboratory of Clinical Studies, Division of Intramural Clinical and Biological Research, National Institute on Alcohol Abuse and Alcoholism, NIH Clinical Center, Bldg. 10, Rm. 3C218, Bethesda, MD 20892.

Reprint requests should be sent to T. Shingu.

jor polyunsaturated fatty acid in the brain.[2] We hypothesized that alcohol might stimulate the metabolism of this polyunsaturated fatty acid to enzymatically oxygenated, biologically active products. We therefore began to examine rat brain for the capacity to produce such products both *in vitro* and *in vivo*.

METHODS

22:6w3 metabolism by rat brain in vitro. Male Sprague-Dawley rats weighing 250-300 g were decapitated and the brains were removed and homogenized in 50 mM tris buffer at pH 7.4. Following a 10-minute preincubation at 37°C, 25 uM [C-14]-22:6w3 was incubated with 1 ml of a 10% homogenate (w/v) for 15 min at 37°C. Formic acid was added in order to terminate the reaction and bring the pH to 3.5. Butylated hydroxy toluene (BHT) was added in order to prevent autooxidation. The incubation mixture was then extracted twice with equal volumes of dichloromethane. The extracts were evaporated under nitrogen, dissolved in methanol and analyzed by reversed phase HPLC. The HPLC conditions were as follows: (a) 5 micron Axxichrom ODS column of 2.6 mm × 25 cm (b) a mobile phase of acetonitrile and 0.1 M ammonium acetate, pH 7.0, (c) the eluant was run at 1 ml/min through a diode array UV detector at both 235 and 280 nm and then into a radioactivity detector. For characterization of the products by rat brain, purified 15- and 5-lipoxygenases were incubated with [C-14]-22:6w3 and the products were analyzed by HPLC under the same condition. Enzyme inhibitors such as 5,8,11,14-eicosatetraynoic acid (ETYA, 0.1uM), caffeic acid (10uM), nordihydroguaiaretic acid (NDGA, 40uM) and indomethacin (10uM) were preincubated with the brain homogenate.

22:6w3 metabolism by rat brain in vivo. Male Sprague-Dawley rats weighing 250-300 g were lightly anesthetized with chloral hydrate and 180 nanomoles of [C-14]-22:6w3 was injected into the left lateral ventricle using a stereotaxic apparatus. After 2 hours, rats were decapitated and the brains rapidly excised. The brain was homogenized in methanol containing BHT. The extract was diluted with methanol to make a 10% solution and applied to a 4 ml Supelco LC-18 cartridge. The ethyl acetate eluant was dried under nitrogen and dissolved in methanol for HPLC analysis. The HPLC conditions were as described above.

22:6w3 metabolism by platelet in vitro. Fresh human venous blood was washed twice with saline containing EDTA (0.01M) and platelets were incubated in 0.2 M tris-HCl, pH 7.5 (0.01M EDTA) with 70 ug of [C-14]-22:6w3 for 20 minutes at 37°C. Formic acid was added in order to terminate the reaction and bring the pH to 3.5. BHT was then added in order to prevent further oxidation. The incubation mixture was extracted twice with equal volumes of dichloromethane, and the extracts were evaporated and dissolved in methanol for analysis by reversed phase HPLC as described above.

Assignment of the structure of 22:6w3 products formed by platelet. The two major metabolites of 22:6w3 formed by platelet were separated by reversed phase HPLC, methylated, trimethylsilylated and analyzed with GC/MS. The structures thus assigned were 11- and 14-hydroxy docosahexaenoates (HDHE).

Biological effects of HDHE. Airway (guinea pig lung parenchyma strip), vascular (rat aortic ring) and visceral (rat stomach strip) smooth muscle preparations were mounted in 40 ml baths in order to investigate the effects of HDHE on baseline smooth muscle tone and contractility measured isotonically.

RESULTS

Five major peaks were found in the radiochromatograms obtained from experiments with the rat brain both *in vitro* (Figure 1) and *in vivo*. The retention times of peaks 2 and 4 were consistent with those of 22:6w3 metabolites produced by purified 15- and 5-lipoxygenases, respectively. Human platelets were used as a source of 12-lipoxygenase[3] and the retention time of the major peak produced after incubation with the 22:6w3 corresponded to that of peak 3 in the rat brain chromatogram. Mass spectral analyses (GC/MS/EI) indicated the presence of both 11- and 14-monohydroxy-22:6w3 metabolites. Moreover, ETYA inhibited the production of HDHE by platelet *in vitro* and it also inhibited the production of peak 3 by rat brain *in vitro*. The 5-lipoxygenase inhibitor, caffeic acid (10uM)

22:6w3 LIPOXYGENATION BY RAT BRAIN IN VITRO

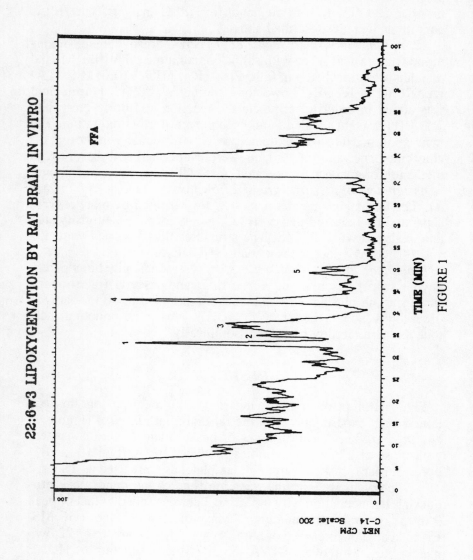

FIGURE 1

238

selectively inhibited the production of peak 4 by 29%. A powerful lipoxygenase inhibitor, NDGA, inhibited the production of all of these compounds at 40uM. The cyclooxygenase inhibitor, indomethacin (10uM), did not affect the production of 22:6w3 metabolites by rat brain *in vitro*.

We report here for the first time that mammalian species are capable of producing oxygenated 22:6w3 metabolites *in vivo*. When [^{14}C]-22:6w3 was injected into the rat lateral ventricle and the brain extracted after 2 hours, all five of the peaks previously observed *in vitro* (Figure 1) were present. A somewhat different distribution of radioactivity among these products was observed with a decrease in the proportion of peak 1 and an increase in that of peaks 3 and 5 observed in the *in vivo* experiment.

Since very little is known about the biological function of these products, an effort was made to explore their potency in smooth muscle systems following purification of the platelet peak by HPLC. A relatively low concentration of HDHE (25 uM) induced a significant increase in the resting tone of both the lung parenchyma and the stomach strip preparations. Resting tension in the rat aortic ring preparation was unaffected. Pretreatment with the lipoxygenase inhibitor, NDGA (40uM), inhibited the HDHE-induced lung parenchymal strip contraction by more than 60%. A cyclooxygenase inhibitor, indomethacin (5 uM) did not significantly alter the contractile response to the HDHE. Consistent with these findings, GC/MS analyses of the lung parenchymal strip incubates collected during the contractile response to HDHE demonstrated no significant change in 2-series prostaglandin levels (PGI2, PXA2, PGE2 and PGF2a). These data may suggest that HDHE induced the release of leukotriene-like substances which contribute to more than 60% of this response. It is not known whether the remaining contractile response observed in the presence of NDGA is a direct effect of HDHE or mediated by other agents. Interestingly, in the preparations studied 25 uM HDHE antagonized the response to U46619 by more than 30%. Preliminary data indicate that 11-HDHE is more efficacious with respect to its contractile and antagonistic effects than the 14-HDHE isomer.

DISCUSSION

This is the first report of HDHE produced *in vivo* in a mammalian species. These products appear to be metabolites of 5-, 12- and 15-lipoxygenases in rat brain and 12-lipoxygenase in human platelet. The 12-lipoxygenase products, monohydroxy docosahexaenoates (HDHE), are present both as 11- and 14-hydroxy docosahexaenoates in the platelet. The HDHE, which was produced by rat brain and platelet *in vitro* when exogenously administered, *induced contraction* in airway and visceral smooth muscle and *antagonized contractility* in all the preparations studied. This contractile effect of HDHE on smooth muscle may be primarily mediated by lipoxygenase but not cyclooxygenase products since NDGA inhibited these responses and indomethacin did not.

REFERENCES

1. Harris RA, Baxter DM, Mitchell MA, Hitzemann RJ. Physical properties and lipid composition of brain membranes from ethanol tolerant-dependent mice. Molecular Pharmac 1984; 25:401-9.

2. Salem Jr. N, Kim H-K, Yergey JA. Docosahexaenoic acid: Membrane function and metabolism. In: Simopoulos AP, Kifer R, Martin RE, eds. Health Effects of Polyunsaturated Fatty Acids in Seafood. New York: Academic Press, 1986:263-317.

3. Aveldano MI, Sprecher H. Synthesis of hydroxy fatty acids from 4,7,10,13,16,19-[1-^{14}C] docosahexaenoic acid by human platelets. J Biol Chem 1983; 258:9339-43.

A New Technique
for Lipid Analysis Using Liquid
Chromatography/Mass Spectrometry

H. Y. Kim, PhD
N. Salem, Jr., PhD

SUMMARY. It has been previously reported that ethanol alters the level of polyunsaturated fatty acids, and this may be related to alteration of membrane physical properties. Therefore, developing a technique to efficiently analyze lipid molecular species is of value for alcohol research.

A new technique which can provide detailed structural information for most major lipid classes has been developed in our laboratory using thermospray liquid chromatography/mass spectrometry (LC/MS). In this technique, on-line LC separation is achieved with a conventional flow rate and the LC effluent is carried into the mass spectrometer via a heated capillary where it is vaporized and ionized. The results thus obtained for the major lipid classes including fast separation methods and quantitative aspects will be presented.

INTRODUCTION

It is generally accepted that ethanol exerts its pharmacological effect through alterations in the physical properties of plasma membranes. These changes including, for example, membrane fluidity may be directly related to the level of polyunsaturated fatty acids esterified to phospholipids. Several reports have shown that ethanol

---

H. Y. Kim and N. Salem, Jr. are affiliated with the Section of Analytical Chemistry, Laboratory of Clinical Studies, Division of Intramural Clinical and Biological Research, National Institute of Alcohol Abuse and Alcoholism, NIH Clinical Center, Bldg. 10, Rm. 3C218, Bethesda, MD 20892.

Reprint requests should be sent to H. Y. Kim.

can alter the levels of polyunsaturates[1,2] but the degree and direction of these changes probably depend upon the ethanol dose, route of administration, duration of exposure, tissue studied and animal species. To evaluate these changes, determination of phospholipid molecular species is required. Nevertheless, the lack of rapid, sensitive and efficient methods for analysis of these compounds has discouraged characterization of biological systems at this level. Recently, a technique for rapid and detailed molecular species analysis of phospholipids was developed in our laboratory using thermospray liquid chromatography/mass spectrometry (LC/MS). Thermospray mass spectrometry is a technique whereby an LC effluent can be introduced directly into a mass spectrometer via a heated capillary interface, thus allowing detection of LC effluents without purification and derivatization.[3] Some of the results obtained by this technique are presented with the fast separation methods newly developed for phospholipid molecular species analysis.

METHODS

The mass spectrometer used in this work was an Extrel ELQ-400 quadrupole system equipped with a standard Vestec thermospray interface. For direct injection, a methanol-0.1M ammonium acetate (95:5) mixture was used as carrier solvent. An electron emitting filament was turned on throughout the experiment to assist ionization.

RESULTS AND DISCUSSION

The typical thermospray spectrum of a phospholipid contains di- and monoglyceride ion peaks resulting from the loss of the phosphoester head group or from the hydrolysis of either fatty acyl moiety from the diglyceride fragment, respectively.[4] In addition, head group ions and intact molecules are also observed. This fragmentation is depicted in Figure 1 for di-16:0-PC. The diglyceride fragment was detected at m/z 552 as the base peak in the spectrum. The monoglyceride ion at m/z 313 and the protonated molecule at m/z 735 provided valuable information as to the fatty acyl composition. The phosphocholine head group was detected at m/z 184 and 142;

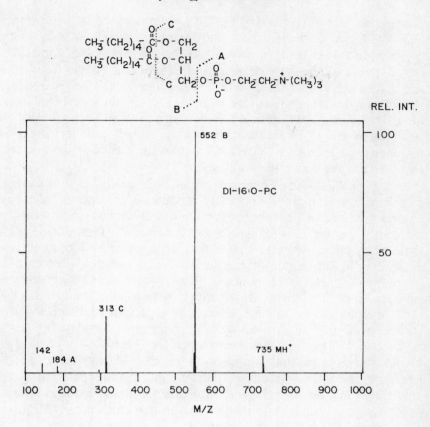

FIGURE 1. Thermospray mass spectrum of di-16:0-PC.

the latter resulted from the loss of trimethylamine from the ammoniated phosphocholine. Therefore, the structure of a phospholipid molecule can be unambiguously assigned by analyzing the spectrum. The same type of fragmentation was observed for phosphatidylethanolamine (PE), phosphatidylserine (PS), phosphatidylinositol (PI), sphingomyelin (SM) and triglycerides.[5] Head group ions distinctive for each class were detected at m/z values of 124, 105 and 198 for PE, PS and PI, respectively. The monoglyceride ion from sphingomyelin resulted from hydrolysis of the amide bond. Platelet activating factor (PAF) generated a similar fragmentation pattern, however, cleavage of the 0-alkyl bond at the sn-1 position was not observed. Since the mass difference in the molecularion or diglyceride fragments with respect to the acylated species are 14 daltons, this species can be readily distinguished on the basis of the thermospray spectra. For the plasmalogens, 0-alkenyl bonds showed easier cleavage than the hydrolysis of the fatty acyl chain at the sn-2 position. The monoglyceride fragment thus formed consti-tuted the base peak in the spectrum. Diglyceride fragments of plas-malogens also showed a characteristic mass difference of 16 daltons compared to the diesterified species.

Using on-line reversed phase chromatography and a hexane: methanol:0.1M ammonium acetate mixture as the mobile phase, natural mixtures of phospholipids were rapidly separated into their molecular species as is shown for bovine liver PI (Figure 2). Five molecular species were separated and detected according to their chain length and degree of unsaturation in 5 minutes. The chro-matographic peaks were assigned by analyzing their thermospray spectra. Since the diglyceride fragments were usually the base peak in the spectra, these ions are selected to represent each species in the reconstructed ion chromatogram. Similarly, fast molecular spe-cies separation methods were developed for other classes of phos-pholipid using methanol:2-propanol:hexane:0.1M ammonium ace-tate mixtures as mobile phase. Phospholipid class separation and detection can also be achieved with this technique using normal phase chromatography and methanol:2-propanol:hexane:0.1M am-monium acetate:acetic acid mixture as the mobile phase.

The absolute amount of particular phospholipid molecular spe-cies could be quantified using calibration curves constructed for each species based on their diglyceride fragments. With selected ion monitoring, linear response curves were obtained in the 0.1 to 10 nmole range for various phosphatidylcholine species when using a column for on-line separation (0.04 to 8 nmole range without a column). These calibration curves were employed to quantify the natural egg-PCs and the results are shown in Table 1. To evaluate this method, fatty acid composition was calculated from the molec-ular species composition data and compared with GC data obtained after transmethylation. The two data sets show good agreement. Some discrepancies were introduced by the species which were not

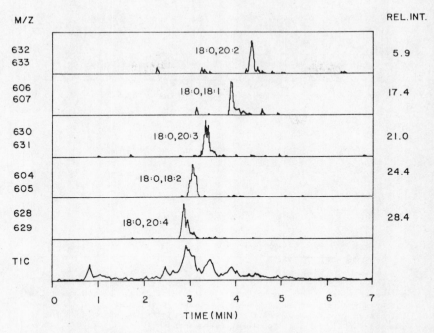

FIGURE 2. Molecular species of bovine liver phosphatidylinositol separated on an Altex Ultrasphere-ODS column (4.6 mm × 7.5 cm) using a mobile phase of methanol:hexane:0.lM ammonium acetate (500:25:30) mixture with a flow rate of 1 mL/min. Diglyceride ions representative of each species are presented with the total ion current (120 to 920 daltons). Relative intensities are shown based on the area percent.

determined by LC/MS since the standards were not available. These results indicate that the quantity of various molecular species can be reliably determined using this method at the subnanomolar level (the detection limit for di-16:0-PC was approximately 20 pmoles). However, this method is only applicable for those species for which standards can be obtained. Alternatively, the relative distribution of various molecular species may provide the information required. With the thermospray technique, this can be readily calculated from the intensities of diglyceride ions obtained in the full mass range scanning mode. The area percentage figures are obtained for the diglyceride ion of each molecular species by dividing its area by the

Table 1. Molecular Species of Egg Phosphatidylcholines

Molecular Species(mol %)[a]		Fatty Acid Composition(wt %)		
16:0, 18:1	34.1		LC/MS[b]	GC[c]
16:0, 18:2	13.8			
18:0, 18:1	5.2	16:0	34.3	31.2
18:1, 18:1	4.5	18:1	36.3	34.4
18:0, 18:2	5.2	18:2	14.2	16.7
16:0, 20:4	2.4	18:0	10.4	13.6
18:0, 20:4	3.5	20:4	4.8	4.1

a. Presented as mole percentages of injected amount (29 nmoles). Only molecular species for which standards were available could be quantified, and they constituted about 69% of total amount injected.
b. Calculated from the molecular species composition and normalized for the composition of the five component fatty acids.
c. Normalized for the composition of the five component fatty acids obtained by GC analysis after transmethylation of egg yolk-PC.

sum of the areas of all the diglyceride peaks detected. This area percent report does not represent the absolute distribution since varying response factors were observed for different species. However, changes in molecular species distribution after pharmacological intervention can still be addressed by comparing the area percentage figures.[6] This approach is now being employed for the study of changes in membrane phospholipid species after ethanol inhalation.

As described above, the thermospray technique can generate both qualitative and quantitative information concerning phospholipid molecular species in a short time. We believe this technique will contribute to alcohol research by facilitating the study of ethanol-induced changes in membrane phospholipid composition and metabolism at the molecular species level.

REFERENCES

1. Littleton JM, John GR, Grieve SJ. Alterations in phospholipid composition in ethanol tolerance and dependence. Alcoholism: Clinical and Experimental Research 1979; 3:50-6.

2. Harris RA, Baxter DM, Mitchell MA, Hitzemann RJ. Physical properties and lipid composition of brain membranes from ethanol tolerant-dependent mice. Mol Pharmacol 1984; 25:401-9.

3. Blakely CR, Vestal ML. Thermospray interface for liquid chromatography/ mass spectrometry. Anal Chem 1983; 55:750-4.

4. Kim HY, Salem Jr. N. Phospholipid molecular species analysis by thermospray LC/MS. Anal Chem 1986; 58:9-14.

5. Kim HY, Salem Jr. N. Application of thermospray high-performance liquid chromatography/mass spectrometry for the determination of phospholipids and related compounds. Anal Chem 1987; 59:722-6.

6. Salem Jr N, Yoffe A, Kim HY, Karanian JW, Taraschi TF. Effects of fish oils and alcohol on polyunsaturated lipids on membranes. In: Lands WEM, ed. Polyunsaturated Fatty Acids and Eicosanoids. Amer Oil Chemists Soc, 1987: 185-91.

SELECTIVE GUIDE TO CURRENT REFERENCE SOURCES ON TOPICS DISCUSSED IN THIS ISSUE

Alcohol Research

Lynn Kasner Morgan, MLS
James E. Raper, Jr., MSLS

Each issue of *Advances in Alcohol & Substance Abuse* features a section offering suggestions on where to look for further information on topics discussed in that issue. In this book, our intent is to guide readers to selected sources of current information on alcohol research.

Some reference sources utilize designated terminology (controlled vocabularies) which must be used to find material on topics of interest. For these a sample of available search terms has been indicated to assist the reader in accessing suitable sources for his/her purposes. Other reference tools use keywords or free-text terms from the title of the document, the abstract, and the name of any responsible agency or conference. In searching using keywords, be sure to look under all possible synonyms to get at the concept in question.

The authors are affiliated with the Gustave L. and Janet W. Levy Library, The Mount Sinai Medical Center, Inc., One Gustave L. Levy Place, New York, NY 10029-6574.

An asterisk (*) appearing before a published source indicates that all or part of that source is in machine-readable form and can be accessed through an online database search. Database searching is recommended for retrieving sources of information that coordinate multiple concepts or subject areas. Most health sciences libraries offer database services or searching can be done from one's office or home with subscriptions to database services and appropriate computer equipment.

Readers are encouraged to consult their librarians for further assistance before undertaking research on a topic.

Suggestions regarding the content and organization of this section are welcome.

1. INDEXING AND ABSTRACTING SOURCES

Place of publication, publisher, start date, frequency of publication, and brief descriptions are noted.

* *Biological Abstracts* (1926-) and *Biological Abstracts/RRM* (v.18, 1980-). Philadelphia, BioSciences Information Service, semimonthly. Reports on worldwide research in the life sciences.
    See: Concept headings for abstracts, such as psychiatry-addiction.
    See: Keyword-in-context subject index.
* *Chemical Abstracts*. Columbus, Ohio, American Chemical Society, 1907- , weekly. A key to the world's literature of chemistry and chemical engineering, including journal articles, patents, reviews, technical reports, monographs, conference proceedings, symposia, dissertations, and books.
    See: *Index Guide* for cross-referencing and indexing policies.
    See: *General Subject Index* terms, such as alcohols; biological studies; drug dependence; drug-drug interactions; drug tolerance.
    See: Keyword subject indexes.
* *Dissertation Abstracts International. Section B. The Sciences and Engineering*. Ann Arbor, MI, University Microfilms, v.30, 1969/70- , monthly. Includes author-prepared abstracts of doctoral dissertations from 500 participating institutions throughout

North America and the world. A separate section contains European dissertations.

See: Keyword-in-context subject index.

* *Excerpta Medica*. Amsterdam, The Netherlands, Excerpta Medica Foundation, 1947 -   , 44 sections. A major abstracting service covering more than 4,500 biomedical journals. The abstracts, including English summaries for non-English-language articles, appear in one or more of the published subject sections, excluding Section 37, *Drug Literature Index*, and Section 38, *Adverse Reactions Titles*, which are indexes only. Each of the sections has a comprehensive subject index. Since 1978 all the *Excerpta Medica* sections have been available for computer searching in the integrated online file EMBASE.

Particularly relevant to the topics in this issue are Section 40, *Drug Dependence*, and the sections that have addiction, alcoholism, or drug subdivisions: Section 30, *Pharmacology*; Section 32, *Psychiatry*; and Section 17, *Public Health, Social Medicine and Hygiene*.

* *Index Medicus*. (including *Bibliography of Medical Reviews*). Bethesda, Md., National Library of Medicine, 1960- , monthly, with annual cumulations. Published as author and subject indexes to more than 2,500 journals in the biomedical sciences. Subject headings are based on the controlled vocabulary or thesaurus, Medical Subject Headings (MeSH). Since 1966 it has been produced from the MEDLARS database, which provides more comprehensive retrieval, including keyword access and English-language abstracts, than its printed counterparts: *Index Medicus*, *International Nursing Index* and *Index to Dental Literature*.

See: *MeSH* terms, such as alcohol drinking; alcohol, ethyl; alcoholic beverages; drug interactions; substance abuse; substance dependence; substance use disorders; substance withdrawal syndrome.

Index to Scientific Reviews. Philadelphia, Institute for Scientific Information, 1974- , semiannual.

See: Permuterm keyword subject index.

See: Citation index.

* *International Pharmaceutical Abstracts*. Washington, D.C., American Society of Hospital Pharmacists, 1964- , semimonthly. A key to the world's literature of pharmacy.

> See: IPA subject terms, such as alcoholism, dependence.

* *Psychological Abstracts*. Washington, D.C., American Psychological Association, 1927- , monthly. A compilation of nonevaluative summaries of the world's literature in psychology and related disciplines.

> See: Index terms, such as addiction, alcohol drinking patterns, alcohol intoxication, alcohol rehabilitation, alcoholic hallucinosis, alcoholic psychosis, alcoholism, drug abuse, drug addiction, drug dependency, drug interactions, drug usage.

* *Public Affairs Information Service Bulletin*. New York, Public Affairs Information Service, v.55, 1969- , semimonthly. An index to library material in the field of public affairs and public policy published throughout the world.

> See: PAIS subject headings, such as alcoholism, drug abuse, drug addicts.

* *Sociological Abstracts*. San Diego, Calif., Sociological Abstracts, Inc., 1952- , 5 times per year. A collection of nonevaluative abstracts which reflects the world's serial literature in sociology and related disciplines.

> See: Descriptors such as alcohol use, alcoholic beverages, alcoholism, drug abuse, drug addiction, drug use, substance abuse.

* *Science Citation Index*. Philadelphia, Institute for Scientific Information, 1961- , bimonthly.

> See: Permuterm keyword subject index.

> See: Citation index.

* *Social Work Research and Abstracts*. New York, National Association of Social Workers, v.13, 1977- , quarterly.

> See: Fields of service sections, such as alcoholism and drug addiction.

> See: Subject index.

2. CURRENT AWARENESS PUBLICATIONS

* *Current Contents: Clinical Medicine*. Philadelphia, Institute for Scientific Information, v.15, 1987- , weekly.
    See: Keyword index.
* *Current Contents: Life Sciences*. Philadelphia, Institute for Scientific Information, v.10, 1967- , weekly.
    See: Keyword index.
* *Current Contents: Social & Behavioral Sciences*. Philadelphia, Institute for Scientific Information, v.6, 1974- , weekly.
    See: Keyword index.

3. BOOKS

Andrews, Theodora. *A Bibliography of Drug Abuse, Including Alcohol and Tobacco*. Littleton, Colo., Libraries Unlimited, 1977- .

Andrews, Theodora. *Guide to the Literature of Pharmacy and the Pharmaceutical Sciences*. Littleton, Colo., Libraries Unlimited, 1986.

* *Medical and Health Care Books and Serials in Print: An Index to Literature in the Health Sciences*. New York, R. R. Bowker Co., annual.
    See: Library of Congress subject headings, such as alcohol, alcoholics, alcoholism, drug abuse, pharmacology, toxicology.

* *National Library of Medicine Current Catalog*. Bethesda, Md., National Library of Medicine, 1966- , quarterly, with annual cumulations.
    See: *MeSH* terms as noted in Section 1 under *Index Medicus*.

4. U.S. GOVERNMENT PUBLICATIONS

* *Monthly Catalog of United States Government Publications*. Washington, D.C., U.S. Government Printing Office, 1895- , monthly.
    See: Following agencies: Alcohol, Drug Abuse and Mental

Health Administration; National Institute of Mental Health; National Institute on Drug Abuse.
See: Subject headings, derived chiefly from the Library of Congress, such as alcohol, alcoholics, alcoholism, drug abuse, drug utilization, drugs, pharmacology, toxicology.
See: Title keyword index.

5. ONLINE BIBLIOGRAPHIC DATABASES

Only those databases which have no print equivalents are included in this section. Print sources which have online database equivalents are noted throughout this guide by the asterisk (*) which appears before the title. If you do not have direct access to these databases, consult your librarian for assistance.

ASI: AMERICAN STATISTICS INDEX (Congressional Information Services, Inc., Washington, D.C.).
Use: Keywords.
DRUG INFO/ALCOHOL USE/ABUSE (Hazelden Foundation, Center City, Minn., and Drug Information Service Center, College of Pharmacy, University of Minnesota, Minneapolis, Minn.).
Use: Keywords.
MAGAZINE INDEX (Information Access Co., Belmont, Calif.).
Use: Keywords.
MEDICAL AND PSYCHOLOGICAL PREVIEWS: MPPS (BRS Bibliographic Retrieval Services, Inc., Latham, N.Y.).
Use: Keywords.
MENTAL HEALTH ABSTRACTS (IFI/Plenum Data Co., Alexandria, Va.).
Use: Keywords.
NATIONAL NEWSPAPER INDEX (Information Access Co., Belmont, Calif.).
Use: Keywords.
NTIS (National Technical Information Service, U.S. Dept. of Commerce, Springfield, Va.).
Use: Keywords.

PSYCALERT (American Psychological Association, Washington, D.C.).

Use: Keywords.

6. HANDBOOKS, DIRECTORIES, GRANT SOURCES, ETC.

Annual Register of Grant Support. Wilmette, Ill., National Register Pub. Co., annual.

See: Medicine; pharmacology; psychiatry, psychology, mental health sections.

See: Subject index.

Directory of Research Grants. Phoenix, Az., Oryx Press. Annual.

See: Subject index terms, such as alcoholism, drug abuse.

* *Encyclopedia of Associations*. Detroit, Gale Research Co., annual (occasional supplements between editions).

See: Subject index.

Encyclopedia of Information Systems and Services. 8th ed. Detroit, Gale Research Co., c1988.

* *Foundation Directory*. New York, The Foundation Center, biennial (updated between editions by *Foundation Directory Supplement*).

See: Index of foundations.

See: Index of foundations by state and city.

See: Index of donors, trustees, and administrators.

See: Index of fields of interest.

Research Awards Index. Bethesda, Md., National Institutes of Health, Division of Research Grants, annual.

See: Subject index.

O'Brien, Robert and Sidney Cohen. *The Encyclopedia of Drug Abuse*. New York, Facts on File Pub., 1984.

Roper, Fred W. and Jo Anne Boorkman. *Introduction to Reference Sources in the Health Sciences*. 2nd ed. Chicago, Medical Library Association, c1984.

7. JOURNAL LISTINGS

* *Ulrich's International Periodicals Directory*. New York, R. R. Bowker Co., annual (updated between editions by *Ulrich's Quarterly*).

   See: Subject categories, such as drug abuse and alcoholism, medical sciences, pharmacy and pharmacology.

8. AUDIOVISUAL PROGRAMS

* *National Library of Medicine Audiovisuals Catalog*. Bethesda, Md., National Library of Medicine, 1977- , quarterly, with annual cumulations.

   See: *MeSH* terms as noted in Section 1 under *Index Medicus*.

Patient Education Sourcebook. [St. Louis, Mo.], Health Sciences Communications Association, c1985.

   See: *MeSH* terms as noted in Section 1 under *Index Medicus*.

9. GUIDES TO UPCOMING MEETINGS

Scientific Meetings. San Diego, Calif., Scientific Meetings Publications, quarterly.

   See: Subject indexes.

   See: Association listing.

World Meetings: Medicine. New York, Macmillan Pub. Co., quarterly.

   See: Keyword index.

   See: Sponsor directory and index.

World Meetings: Outside United States and Canada. New York, Macmillan Pub. Co., quarterly.

   See: Keyword index.

   See: Sponsor directory and index.

World Meetings: United States and Canada. New York, Macmillan Pub. Co., quarterly.

   See: Keyword index.

   See: Sponsor directory and index.

10. PROCEEDINGS OF MEETINGS

* *Conference Papers Index*. Louisville, Ky., Data Courier, v.6, 1978- , monthly.
Directory of Published Proceedings. Series SEMT. Science/Engineering/Medicine/Technology. White Plains, N.Y., InterDok Corp., v.3, 1967- , monthly, except July-August, with annual cumulations.
* *Index to Scientific and Technical Proceedings*. Philadelphia, Institute for Scientific Information, 1978- , monthly with semiannual cumulations.

11. SPECIALIZED RESEARCH CENTERS

Medical Research Centres. 7th ed. Harlow, Essex, Longman, 1986.
International Research Centers Directory. 4th ed. Detroit, Gale Research Co., 1988-89, c1988.
Research Centers Directory. 12th ed. Detroit, Gale Research Co., 1988 (updated by *New Research Centers*).

12. SPECIAL LIBRARY COLLECTIONS

Ash, L., comp. *Subject Collections*. 6th ed. New York, R. R. Bowker Co., 1985.
Directory of Special Libraries and Information Centers. 11th ed. Detroit, Gale Research Co., 1988 (updated by *New Special Libraries*).